LIVING WITH
SCHIZOPHRENIA

PSYCHOLOGICAL DISORDERS SERIES

Court and *Nelson,* Bipolar Puzzle Solution: A Mental Health Client's Perspective.
Emmons, Geiser, Kaplan, and *Harrow,* Living with Schizophrenia.

LIVING WITH SCHIZOPHRENIA

Stuart Emmons
Craig Geiser
Kalman Kaplan, Ph.D.
Martin Harrow, Ph.D.

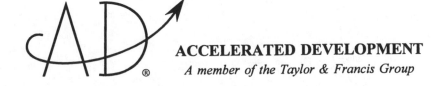

ACCELERATED DEVELOPMENT
A member of the Taylor & Francis Group

USA	Publishing Office:	ACCELERATED DEVELOPMENT
		A member of the Taylor & Francis Group
		1101 Vermont Avenue, N.W., Suite 200
		Washington, DC 20005-3521
		Tel: (202) 289-2174
		Fax: (202) 289-3665
	Distribution Center:	ACCELERATED DEVELOPMENT
		A member of the Taylor & Francis Group
		1900 Frost Road, Suite 101
		Bristol, PA 19007-1598
		Tel: (215) 785-5800
		Fax: (215) 785-5515
UK		Taylor & Francis Ltd.
		1 Gunpowder Square
		London EC4A 3DE
		Tel: 071 405 2237
		Fax: 071 831 2035

LIVING WITH SCHIZOPHRENIA

1 2 3 4 5 6 7 8 9 0   B R B R   9 8 7

This book was set in Times Roman. The editors were Heather Worley and Cynthia Long. Cover design by Michelle Fleitz.

A CIP catalog record for this book is available from the British Library.
∞ The paper in this publication meets the requirements of the ANSI Standard Z39.48-1984 (Permanence of Paper)

Library of Congress Cataloging-in-Publication Data

Living with schizophrenia / Stuart Emmons, Craig Geiser ; Kalman
    Kaplan, Martin Harrow.
       p.   cm.
    Includes bibliographical references.

    1. Emmons, Stuart.   2. Geiser, Craig.   3. Schizophrenics–
Biography.   4. Schizophrenia.   I. Emmons, Stuart.   II. Geiser,
Craig.   III. Kaplan, Kalman J.   IV. Harrow, Martin.
RC514.L573   1997
616.89'82'00922—dc21
[B]   97-19055
                                                                            CIP

ISBN 1-56032-566-9 (paper)

Throughout this book, names of people and places have been changed.

CONTENTS

PREFACE

Several years ago, we first encountered the personal accounts of Stuart and Craig regarding their experiences with schizophrenia. We were moved by their stories and were touched by their artistry. A number of Stuart's poems are very poignant; Craig's cartoons provide a very sharp relief. We felt that these works represented important documents in our encounter with mentally ill patients. It was important, we felt, for the general public to understand these patients' lives as they themselves did—in other words, to provide an *inside* view of the lives of people living with and suffering from schizophrenia. This seemed especially important to us in a modern world where the sick and elderly often are portrayed from the *outside* as having poor, unremittingly miserable existences.

Such a superficial approach to the mentally ill is objectionable on many grounds. First, these outside descriptions often are made cavalierly without any real understanding of the fabric of the patients' day-to-day lives. This serves to discount real achievements that people who are mental patients may make and serves to deprive them of a genuine source of self-esteem. Second, these outside descriptions tend to deprive them of any hope of improvement, tending to evoke a downward spiraling cycle—the more hopeless they are, the more depressed and even suicidal they may become. We often have observed in our own research and in our individual treatment of schizophrenia patients the occurrence of secondary depression in schizophrenia as schizophrenia patients become aware that they might not achieve many of the life goals they had set for themselves prior to the onset of their illness. Third, this negative view of mental patients may serve to isolate these people from "healthy society," leading others to stigmatize them as "only patients" rather than as people and attempting to dehumanize them. Such a view is potentially very dangerous in an era of shrinking health resources and debates about euthanasia. Some might want to choose what seems like an easy path and "write off" the mentally ill as being either sick or unproductive. The first description portrays the patient as an unfortunate *victim* who has a poor "quality of life." The second description paints the same patient as draining *victimizer* who has become "too costly to keep alive," whether in emotional or financial terms.

The accounts of Stuart and Craig are important because they make it impossible for the general public to simply dismiss them as "schizophrenics" or "patients." These accounts provide compelling portraits of "full people" who have dealt with schizophrenia in their lives, sometimes unsuccessfully (typically early in their disease), but often quite successfully (later in the course of their illness). We feel their confusion and at times cry with them. We rejoice in their recovery and laugh with them. We admire their insight and realize that like them, we all have talents we should develop, and limitations and disabilities we must work to overcome.

We are honored to participate in this project, offering professional insight into the lives of Stuart and Craig, while simultaneously affirming our view of them as people with dreams and disappointments and the capacity for resiliency. Our expertise and experience allow us to begin to recognize important symptomatic patterns that may occur for many people who live with schizophrenia. Our approach to Stuart and Craig also emphasizes the struggle of two very courageous people trying to make "something" of their lives. We all can learn from this and from them.

Kalman J. Kaplan, Ph.D., & Martin Harrow, Ph.D.

INTRODUCTION

Note: Throughout this text, all comments from Dr. Kaplan and Dr. Harrow, psychologists, are presented in indented and *italicized* print, preceded by the letters **PN:** (Psychologists' Note).

Craig Geiser and I (Stuart Emmons), paranoid schizophrenics, first met in group therapy. Over time, each discovered that the other had written about his schizophrenic experiences. In addition, Craig showed me pictures of faces he drew to express his feelings. Subsequently, we decided to merge our work and develop this book, which is based on our views of schizophrenia from the standpoint of two people who have experienced it, along with professional comments of Doctors Kalman Kaplan and Martin Harrow, two mental health professionals and university professors who have treated schizophrenia patients, have conducted extensive research on schizophrenia, and have written about it.

Our stories clearly illustrate the strange and frightening world of the paranoid schizophrenic. But, strangely, we also found that world both exciting and awesome. Thinking of our experiences as adventures, we decided to entitle our book *Living with Schizophrenia*. The action in these adventures comes fast. A staggering number of thoughts enter one's mind. In fact, it is amazing that Craig and I were able to sort the thoughts out and come up with an accurate description. I find it surprising that I can remember so clearly ideas that happened almost two decades ago. While Craig's memories are of more recent experiences, it still is incredible how vividly he can remember these things when they were so confusing at the time.

It should be emphasized that Craig and I, by using medication, appear quite normal now. Unless there is a medical breakthrough, however, we always will be diagnosed as paranoid schizophrenics.

In "A Peculiar Time," I write about when I was in a state mental hospital. In "My World: The Evening Years," I write about my present condition and about when I was actively ill in my story. While my hospitalization occurred some time ago, I understand from people who have been in the hospital recently that conditions are much the same as when I was there, except that there aren't nearly as many patients there now.

Craig has drawn pictures of faces—especially through the eyes—that express his feelings and that are an interesting, unique presentation of a schizophrenic's perceptions.

We hope that you enjoy this book for what it is—an attempt to record interesting experiences. While neither Craig nor I ever would wish anybody to go through the schizophrenic experience, it is an exciting view of reality, the schizophrenic reality, and it ought to be more understood by the general public.

You might wonder, what is schizophrenia? Craig says this, "When someone asks me to explain schizophrenia, I tell them I have a way of making them understand it. I tell them, 'You know how sometimes you are in your dreams yourself, and some of them feel like real nightmares?' Most people can relate to this. Then, I tell them, 'It was like I was walking through a dream but everything around me was real.' At times, today's world seems so boring and I wonder if I would like to step back into the schizophrenic dream, but then I remember all the scary and horrifying experiences.

> **PN:** *From the perspective of the experienced mental health professionals who are participating in this joint project, we can note that Stuart is thinking, in part, about altered states of consciousness. Whether or not schizophrenia represents an altered state of consciousness has been debated back and forth for decades (Bowers, 1974). Currently, most professionals do not feel that schizophrenia represents an altered state of consciousness, and we also do not feel that the essence of schizophrenia is an altered state of consciousness. This is still an open issue, however, that has not been completely resolved.*

Craig and I started writing this book in an attempt to help cope with our past experiences by writing about and defining them. Craig writes, "I wanted to put all of my schizophrenic experiences into order so that while talking to someone about it, I wouldn't have a staggered, jumbled-up explanation. It's like having a jigsaw puzzle in your head and trying to put the last pieces into place. When your last piece is found and put in its proper place, there is such an overwhelming relief and satisfaction. I wanted to straighten out this great mystery, schizophrenia. For when I first heard I was schizophrenic, I thought, schizophrenia, me, why me, what is schizophrenia?"

Like Craig, I marvel at my schizophrenic experiences. I found them painful but now, as memories, precious for the vivid feelings they gave me.

Craig and I have come to a recognition that there are few opportunities for health professionals, relatives of paranoid schizophrenics, and the public at large to understand the disease up close. Thus, we are writing the book, not only for its interest, but for how it might contribute to an inside-outside look at the disease.

We conclude this introduction with questions we answered that were given to us recently in a psychology class at August College.

QUESTIONS ASKED CRAIG

1. When you started hearing voices for the second time, had your medication been changed recently?

During my second admittance to the hospital, my medication hadn't been changed recently, but I had been taken off my medicine for approximately one year while I attended the rehabilitation center.

2. In your comments, you mentioned that you had to ask what your disorder was. When you discovered what it was, you had misconceptions of it. Do you believe educating those with behavior disorders would be helpful?

I feel that it would be extremely helpful to have a name to go along with my disorder and educating me would have me accept it while making me a whole human being and able to interact with an understanding and self-worth.

3. It has been found that certain behavior traits develop prior to a relapse. Did you realize when you were relapsing?

Both times in becoming mentally ill, I had an inner feeling things were not right in my head. The first and second time I sought out a person as a safeguard.

PN: *We can note that the issue of whether schizophrenia patients are aware of their difficulties when they are becoming more severely psychotic or having a psychotic "break" is a tricky issue. At the time of a psychotic "break," many people lose perspective about whether they are beginning to behave in a socially inappropriate manner. Their self-monitoring, which is based in part on the effective use of stored knowledge or long-term memory, becomes poorer (Harrow, Lanin-Kettering, & Miller, 1989). Thus, at the very time when good monitoring or adequate perspective is most needed to request more medication or to request being put on medication if they are not on it at the time, the potentially psychotic patients are not completely aware of their difficulty. In the one period when judgment about getting extra treatment is most needed, many patients are least able to show good judgment in this area. Many, but not all, schizophrenia patients show poor monitoring of their own difficulties at the time when they begin to become psychotic (Benson & Stuss, 1990; Frith, 1995; Frith & Done, 1988; Harrow et al., 1989; Harrow & Miller, 1980; Port, Harrow, Jobe & Dougherty, in press).*

4. How did you meet your wife? What was her reaction to your illness?

I met my wife through the jobs we possessed together in a nursing home. She had known about schizophrenia through previous encounters on the job before dating one another.

5. Was there any reason why most of your artwork was done in 1984? Where were you during that year?

Most of my artwork had taken place during 1984 while working night shift at the nursing home. It was a scapegoat for relaxation to relieve the tension of my new career.

6. Didn't it even seem strange that people were dying right outside your hospital door?

I was letting my mind control my thoughts of hallucinating delusions of people dying outside my doorway at the hospital.

7. Did you ever want to help them?

I wanted so much to help each and every one of them but I knew that if I was to sacrifice myself that all I stood for to them would be ruined.

8. When you look back on your hallucinations, do they seem as though they really occurred even though you knew they were hallucinations or do they seem like bad dreams?

Really occurred. Very frightening.

9. What are some of the differences between your marriage and that of a marriage without schizophrenia?

Just have to work it out and be supportive.

10. Is there a difference between your drawings when you are in a state of confusion and when you are not?

While drawing before the schizophrenia, I was not as creative as I am now.

> **PN:** *Let us discuss the relationship between schizophrenia and creativity. This issue has been controversial for over a century. Many romantic observers have proposed that schizophrenia patients are more "creative" than people without psychiatric problems. As of yet, there is no solid evidence for this. Almost in contrast, Andreasen has presented evidence linking people with affective disorders, or mood disorders, and creativity (Andreasen & Powers, 1974, 1975). Andreasen's evidence about a link between creativity and mood disorders seems quite strong. It should not be forgotten, however, that many people without mental disorders, such as "normals," are quite creative, as are select people with schizophrenia, such as Stuart and Craig.*

11. Do you still think about Bob Seger's song, "Still the Same," and does it hold the same meaning, if any, for you today?

Bob Seger's song has a lot of the same feeling to me today as it meant to me back in 1978.

12. During the time you are not in a hospital, do you practice any kind of self-therapy like the exercises you did in groups you were in while you were hospitalized?

I still do one of the exercises I had learned when in the hospital. The one on relaxation is very helpful in many ways, such as that it brings out the most comfortable and refreshing feeling to my whole body and mind.

13. Because you are conscious of the fact that you have schizophrenia, are you aware when you're having schizophrenic episodes and, if so, how often do you have them?

I was somewhat aware both times prior to being admitted to the hospital, but there are times when I begin to wonder and worry that maybe I'm going back into that state.

14. Do you have any family members who have or have had schizophrenia?

As far as I understand, there isn't any schizophrenia in my family background.

15. Do you think it's worth it to take the medicine even with the side effects?

Yes, I think it is very beneficial to take your medicine along with some type of counseling. The side effects from my medication are no problem for me to cope with. I think it would be very beneficial for the physician to explain all the side effects with their patients.

16. What type of therapy are you in currently?

The therapy for me right now is writing, drawing, and working on getting this book published to help others deal with the understanding of schizophrenia and the schizophrenic.

17. When you were in the hospital with delusions and hallucinations, did any of the words of your family and the doctors get through?

For quite some time, there was great resentment and frustration towards both family members and doctors because I didn't believe they understood what was going on in my head. I thought they were all crazy and needed a lot more help than me.

18. Did the hallucinations and delusions come on all of a sudden?

The hallucinations and delusions did seem to come on all of a sudden from my point of view. The voices began bombarding me from all directions. I knew deep inside there was a great disbelief and an onset of confusion that could not be handled solely by myself.

19. Do you think the media (including movies and television) had much effect on the subject matter of your hallucinations and delusions?

At one point, there was a movie that the special effects seemed so real to me that I thought this was a live broadcast of what was actually happening. I didn't tell anyone for fear that this torture might happen to me.

20. Is the illness totally controlled by your medication?

I don't think my medication is totally controlling the illness. I think that it is a combination of myself wanting to get better with the help of a variety of one-to-one interaction.

> **PN:** *From our perspective, it seems clear that anti-psychotic medication and treatment in general can help, and indeed do help the majority of patients with schizophrenia. Thus, the anti-psychotic medications shorten acute episodes, diminish their intensity, and probably avoid some episodes, but not all of them. Thus, people with schizophrenia, even in the best of treatment, are still vulnerable to potential psychosis and other symptoms associated with this illness (Breier, Schrieber, Dyer, & Pickar, 1991; Harrow, MacDonald, Sands, & Silverstein, 1995; Harrow, Sands, Silverstein, & Goldberg, in press; Johnstone, 1990; McGlashan, 1984; Tsuang & Fleming, 1987). The medications have not cured schizophrenia, and there are still many disordered schizophrenia patients although a large number are less disordered than they once would have been prior to the discovery of modern neuroleptics and other newer anti-psychotic medications. Thus, it is important to observe that Craig is correct here and that an important factor in clinical improvement for people with schizophrenia is that they themselves try to work towards bettering themselves, trying to keep calm and controlled, trying to keep a positive attitude, and trying to use their abilities as best they can.*

21. Did people treat you differently after they found out you had schizophrenia?

I usually had to explain to them what schizophrenia was, but I don't think they treated me any differently once they found out what I was really like.

22. Is it difficult now to accept the hallucinations as not real when they at the time seemed so real?

It is very difficult to accept the hallucinations as not real when they did seem so real at the time. One of the best ways I've found in clarifying it clearly for myself was in obtaining my hospital files. It's like having my own personal diary of the day-by-day reports of me. I thought schizophrenics were wild and possessed people who should be locked up in insane asylums.

QUESTIONS ASKED STUART

1. Was commitment to Christ real or just part of the paranoia?

When I thought I was poisoned, I really did become committed to Christ to find out what happened to me and to have faith no matter what had happened to me.

2. How did the disease affect family members?

All the members of my family were supportive.

3. How did the hospital aid in healing other than administering drugs?

All the hospitals I was in believed in treating the whole person and had therapy programs in addition to medication.

4. How should a person respond to a person who hears voices and gives an explanation of where the voices are from?

You cannot argue with such a person, so just hear them out.

5. Before your initial onset, would you describe yourself as being dependent or independent?

I was very independent and becoming more independent each day.

6. Have your friends become mentally ill, or have you just lost old friends and the new ones are mentally ill?

I just lost old friends and the new ones are mentally ill.

7. How do you and Craig feel about each other? Do you really trust each other? Do you often talk deep?

Craig and I trust each other. We both feel we communicate with each other on a deep level through our book. We live a good distance apart, so we don't talk often.

8. How are you treated today when someone is told you are schizophrenic?

One woman told me I was possessed by demons, but most people are friendly, but curious.

9. What was your childhood like?

I had a wonderful, normal childhood.

10. Any schizophrenic signs in childhood?

No, but in the 10th grade I got an ulcer, saw a psychiatrist, and was put on tranquilizers.

11. Stuart, in your poems, you talked about loving and being loved. Does that make a difference?

Yes, love is what is needed most.

12. Do your poems work as an outlet for you as well as the drawings for Craig?

Yes, I would say the creativity involved is an outlet for both of us where we can express ourselves.

> **PN:** *Again, from our viewpoint, we can observe that being able to do things for oneself and to succeed enhances ones self-image. This can lead to a better outlook, lead to more satisfaction, and improve one's own mental condition, although nothing is foolproof.*

13. Was it difficult to write the book and did it bring up memories of the past?

It was a thrill to write the book. It was at times dealing with painful memories. But they also seemed to be precious memories.

14. Do you continue to write poetry? And do you find it therapeutic?

Yes, I still write poetry, and I do find it therapeutic. I have written a collection of poems about when I was in General State Hospital entitled *A Sensitive Time.* I also wrote a collection of poems about when I was actively mentally ill in the last half of the 1960s. It is entitled *The Twilight Years.*

15. Stuart, you mentioned that while in the mental hospital, you were misunderstood, no matter what you did. Is this a continuing source of frustration even today?

No. Today, fortunately, I feel I am understood. The only misunderstanding I come across is when people think I am a lot different than they are.

16. What role does your faith play?

I feel Christ is the only one who knows what is really going on, that he understands me and can direct me. When I was actively ill, I thought Christ could understand me, because he too knew what it meant to be misunderstood. But while I was misunderstood for not knowing what was going on, Christ was misunderstood because he was the only one who knew what was going on.

> **PN:** *From our vantage point, Stuart's distinction is very interesting. Stuart acknowledges that when he was actively ill, he "didn't know what was going on," so in what sense was he misunderstood? Stuart identifies with his image of Christ who he feels was "the only one who knew what was going on." In other words, Stuart tries to distinguish two ways in which a person can be misunderstood—either by being sicker than others or by being healthier than others. This represents a very subtle curvilinear view of mental health and social adjustment. The best social adjustment occurs for people of moderate mental health. The question remains as to what does this view add to Stuart's sense of well-being?*

17. What kinds of situations do you encounter with other people in day-to-day life?

I find I am understood quite well by others. I live a normal life now, just like anyone else.

STUART'S STORY

In the winter of 1965, having graduated from August College *cum laude*, I began doing graduate work at Green University near Detroit. I had signed up for six courses of graduate work and was prepared, I thought, for a successful semester that would lead to a career in community college teaching.

My mother and father put a second mortgage on our family home in Lake City, MI, to provide the money for college. I was sure that within a year I would be teaching in a community college and be paying back the loan.

When my parents drove me to campus, I was scared. This was to be my first time away from them. They parked the car in front of Jason Hall, an older three-story brick structure. I found my room on the third floor. This was a time when colleges were overloaded with students. To my amazement, my two-man room would be home for three students.

> **PN:** *From the mental health framework, what is important is that Stuart indicates that this is the first time he would be away from his parents.*

The room contained one large desk with a chair and drawers on each side. Two chairs for three students! The bedroom had three beds, two of which were bunk beds. Being the nice guy, I agreed to take the upper bed, and I even let my roommates have the bedroom window open when it was snowing out. I became terribly sick and slept with my clothes on and got better in 24 hours. One of my roommates got pneumonia.

1

I was very busy though I was happy. I studied until 11:00 every night. I liked going to a little restaurant for coffee in the morning, but other than that I didn't waste much time. On weekends, one of my dorm mates took me in his car to a nearby city for lunch. Occasionally, we went out with another graduate student, Steve Dunn.

I learned that there was a vacant room in Jason Hall, Room 13. I applied for and soon received it. I asked my roommates to help me move my possessions, but they said they were busy. So I moved my belongings as quickly as I could by myself. The room was a single, with a desk and bed in it, and I felt privileged to get it. It was a basement room next to a large dormitory study room.

   PN: *Note that Stuart moves to a vacant room to elude problems.*

Strange things were beginning to happen. In the dining hall, a girl came up to me and asked me why, on the previous day, I had asked her not to sit next to me. I couldn't remember. And I had a strange desire to wear a red pullover shirt with a sport suit.

As the warmer weather of spring came, my room became very warm. Then I actually had bugs crawling on the floor, and I was horrified. The bugs multiplied rapidly and were on the floor day after day. I was becoming nervous and called a friend on the telephone. He suggested that I relax and listen to music on the radio. But I had loaned my radio to one of my former roommates, and I was convinced that he was listening to me on it.

   PN: *For Stuart, paranoia begins with real bugs but then moves to feelings of being listened to on the radio ("being bugged"). So, in one sense Stuart can distinguish between real and imagined "bugs."*

One night I was invited to listen to a foreign service official talk. I was suspicious of him and thought he thought I was a Communist spy. I didn't say anything. I just stared at him.

   PN: *We note here the beginning of the psychotic experience. It is facilitated by Stuart's feeling anxious and uncertain, with this process accelerated by his being away from his familiar setting (see Bowers, 1974). It is unlikely that these heightened pressures, Stuart's feeling of anxiety, and his heightened cognitive arousal alone account for this psychotic break, but in a vulnerable person such as Stuart, they are probably contributors.*

One night I went to the shower room but found myself locked out of my room and I had forgotten the key. The next day I lost my key and had to get another one to get in my room. I was getting more and more nervous. I was asked if I forgot to bring the broom back to the office after cleaning my room. I thought they thought that I had stolen it.

> **PN:** *Note that Stuart is beginning to lose things—keys, etc.*

The bugs continued to crawl on the floor. I thought the Government was spying into my room with a telescope in a building across the street. I thought people in the cafeteria were loading my food down with salt. In criminology class, I thought the professor and the other students were laughing about me and directing the poisoning of my food in the cafeteria. I managed to live in spite of the poison. When I went to the cafeteria, my hand shook as the girl poured what I thought was poisonous coffee into my cup. I thought everyone in the cafeteria knew I was going to die. They all thought it was too bad, but I was so evil it was necessary.

> **PN:** *Again, one can see how the strange psychotic ideas have increased, have amplified and become stranger, and for the moment have become the dominant factor in Stuart's life. He deserves to be poisoned because he is so evil.*

On a Saturday, I drank lemonade to try to neutralize the poison. Then I would take showers to try to sweat the poison out. I was so nervous I could hardly think. I thought I might only have hours left to live. I thought of taking a bus home to my parents. But no, it was too late for that.

> **PN:** *Note Stuart is coherent enough to try to neutralize the "poison" in a somewhat reasonable way—through drinking lemonade.*

> *One might attempt to understand reality distortions and delusions using the construct of the paranoid pseudo-community developed years ago by Cameron (Cameron, 1963; Cameron & Margaret, 1951). In part, the person or patient has constructed a paranoid pseudo-community, which involves a reconstruction of reality involving some real and at times imagined persons into a conspiracy with the person or patient as the focus of the action.*

> *The paranoid pseudo-community is not a completely false world that the person, on the subjective level, lives in. Rather, it is a world that is partly based on real people and their real social interaction,*

and partly based on a fantasy world of the patient, with these two worlds interacting. Using this outlook towards a delusional patient, the patient's behavior is based in part on his paranoid pseudo-community and in part on the real world.

We have noted these views about the paranoid pseudo-community at this point in relation to Stuart's reality distortions and delusions. However, this concept can be applied at many points in the narrative of Stuart and Craig about their experiences involving reality distortions.

Saturday night I felt that there was an evil presence in my room on my bed. I dared not lie on the bed or I thought something terrible would happen.

PN: *Note Stuart's fear of an evil presence. He is afraid to be on his bed.*

Then, that night, I did something incredible. With my thinking, I had an intellectual religion; I surrendered my intellect to Jesus. I opened the Bible and read "Be a fool for Christ." That was it, I thought. The only one I could appeal to was Jesus. That night I decided that I would see the administrative head of the dormitory the next day. I would tell him I thought that I was poisoned and wanted to see a doctor. I knew that if I was wrong, I would be considered mentally ill. But I couldn't lose. I would be a fool for Christ.

PN: *Stuart decides to "Surrender [his] intellect to Jesus." He tries to set up a no-lose situation. If he is correct that he is being poisoned, he can stop it. If he is incorrect, he is a "fool for Christ." What is important from a mental health point of view is that Stuart take a traditional Christian image, being a "fool for Christ," and distorts it to fit his mental illness. This often happens in schizophrenia where an image that is common in normal thinking becomes psychotic.*

Even in my paranoia—a word I would soon hear for the first time—I could trust Jesus. It was the turning point in my life. I was turning out from myself, out toward Jesus. I was making him my anchor when I thought I might die. Even in my confusion, I knew He was the only one who really understood me and knew what the truth was.

I knew Jesus was betrayed and knew what it was like when everyone seemed to be against Him. He would understand my situation.

PN: *Stuart develops the delusion that he, like Jesus, was betrayed and misunderstood.*

On Sunday morning, when I looked at a book, I wasn't even able to read. I went to the administrator of the dorm like I had planned. He had two graduate students walk me to the health center. A woman there gave me something to drink and, to my astonishment, I drank it. She offered to have me rest at her home a few days, but I declined. Then the two graduate students drove me a few miles to Grayling to the neuropsychiatric institute at Crown University.

When I got there, a man in a white suit introduced himself as Dr. Black. I knew he was a psychiatrist but, because I could reason, I didn't consider myself insane. He asked me to sign in. I didn't want to, but I had no way to get back to the university that I was attending, so I did. Dr. Black left the room, leaving me alone for a short period. I heard voices coming from the heat vent.

PN: *Note Stuart's clever adaptation of a definition of insanity (being able to reason) that keeps him sane by definition. At the same time, he began to hear a voice coming from the vent.*

I thought that he put a speaker there to fool me. I was then led into a residence hall. I met people there who said "hello" but seemed lethargic. I told Dr. Black that they were just as sane as me. He said that was why I was there. I had always thought that insane people couldn't communicate.

PN: *Stuart again is playing with definitions. "Insane people couldn't communicate." These people can communicate; therefore, they are sane—as sane as him.*

Soon I was in bed. I was offered a pill. I thought that if I took the pill offered me by the small nurse, I would die. But I was terribly tired, and I didn't feel like resisting my fate much longer. Finally, I took the pill, confident I would not wake up the next morning.

The next morning, to my astonishment, I awoke. I knew that I was not poisoned at Green University. I wanted to go back to my studies, but I was told that I must rest. I realized that I was paranoid, that I falsely thought that I had been persecuted.

PN: *Again, we could note that Stuart's "insights" are at least partly correct. As we have noted elsewhere in this book, even people who are psychotic are usually not psychotic in all areas all the time. They have some grasp of reality even while they are psychotic in many areas.*

Now I was convinced that I was better and could not see why I had to be hospitalized.

> **PN:** *For example, Stuart realizes he is not poisoned. He realizes he is paranoid, but he continues to intellectually look for reasons why he doesn't have to be hospitalized.*

But I was still ill. I thought that Dr. Black had chosen his name so that I would realize that he was depressing. I thought that my roommate, Eye Eagle, was a detective and that was why he called himself that. Actually, he was a very kind professor at Crown University who was suffering from the trauma of a recent divorce. Nobody seemed to be mentally ill to me. They were all just people with problems.

> **PN:** *Stuart indicates that he doesn't think other patients are "mentally ill," just people with problems.*

One nice woman patient was a nurse who had been flown in. She told me she had spent a night with a patient who died and it had been too much for her.

It wasn't long before my dad came in. He looked like he had been crying. Still seriously mentally ill, I said, "Pa, I outdid Albert Einstein. I blew up my brains. He just developed the atom bomb." I thought that Dr. Black was listening to us. I thought he had the room bugged.

> **PN:** *Stuart reports imagery of blowing up his brain—he is grandiose—he compares himself with Einstein.*

It was not long before I knew most of the people on my floor of the building. There was the woman who had been in a car accident. There was the janitor too nervous to return to his job. There was the man with amnesia. There was a middle-aged heavyset woman who thought that she was dying from cancer. And there were the two high school students who had been on drugs.

Let me tell you more about the environment. I was in a research center, and my blood was taken once a week. In a few days, I was getting relaxed. There was a movie theater in the building where we saw a movie about a plane that crashed, and the survivors found that they were in a high mountainous land where there was peace and people were wise and lived hundreds of years. There was volleyball and baseball outdoors. We went on a bus a few times to a park on a picnic. There was a crafts room I worked in on my floor. There was a large crafts shop on a different floor where I did painting. There was a gymnasium. We went on walks around the Crown University campus. Everything was dark green. The campus was beautiful. It seemed hard to believe that just a few miles away was the Green University campus where I was following my dreams in graduate school.

We had fruit juice drinks every night. We'd play games and watch television. Then one day I realized I had signed in and I could sign out. I told Dr. Black that I wanted to sign out. He said I could, but that he'd like me to stay two more weeks. I signed out. In a few days, I would be home. I had stayed in the hospital four weeks. I would remember the friends I had made and how Professor Eye Eagle said that my parents loved me.

One warm day I was walking with our group back to the neuropsychiatric building when I saw my parents' car parked by the side of the street. I knew they had come to take me home. I was exhilarated. Sure enough, when I got up to my floor, Mom and Dad were waiting for me. I loved them so much. Dr. Black called me in his office for a moment and told me he hoped that all would go well for me. I felt he was taping what we were saying. Soon, I was out free with my parents.

PN: *Note Stuart's psychosis seems to ease at this point.*

My parents took me back to Jason Hall at Green University to pick up any mail that might have come to me. It was a strange feeling for me walking into the dormitory. The day was Sunday, exam time, with only a few days left in the semester. I saw a number of familiar faces, but the students seemed to avoid me. No one said "hello"; I felt as though they thought that I had done something wrong, that I was untouchable. The only mail I had was a package. But it was priceless. It was my college degree from August College.

Earlier my parents had taken all the things in my dorm room home for me, so all I had to take with me was my diploma. My parents told me that my graduate school professors agreed to let me complete my courses by writing a term paper for each of them.

As he always liked to do, my father took the back highways going home instead of the freeways. It was an enjoyable ride home, and I noticed each high school as a possible place of employment. I wasn't planning to go back to Green University.

I went to the August College placement office, hoping to get a teaching job. They told me that there was an opening in Geral High School in Geral,

MI, a farming community only eight miles or so southeast of Lake City. The job consisted of 11th-grade American history and 10th-grade English composition. I was delighted. I didn't admit on the application that I had been mentally ill. My dad said if I did, they wouldn't hire me. After I applied, I just relaxed, ready to enjoy the summer.

> **PN:** *Note Stuart's work ethic in his ordering of events. First he applies to teach high school, then he is free to enjoy summer. You can do your work first; then you play.*

First, I took a beautiful two-week trip in Canada with my mom and dad. We went along the northern shore of Lake Superior and then to Lake-of-the-Woods. It was a beautiful trip. Then my mother and I went out west for the first time to visit my brother in Long Beach, CA.

My brother was a school teacher who was studying psychology to be a school psychologist. He took us to Disneyland, San Diego, and Hollywood. Going home on the train was beautiful too. But every now and then I thought I saw my brother on the train. I thought, at times, he was secretly coming home with me.

> **PN:** *Note Stuart's hallucinations here.*

Mom and I came in on the train at the Lake City station where Dad was waiting for us. He was drunk. He didn't even ask us if we had a good time. It was a big let down at the end of our journey.

> **PN:** *Upon his return from the trip with Mom, Stuart finds his dad drunk at the train station. Does this reflect Dad's jealousy?*

The summer was going by quickly. In August, I received a call for a job interview with the Superintendent of the Geral schools. I dressed in my black suit and walked into the new high school building to the Superintendent's office. He hired me on the spot. It was 1965, and there was still a teachers shortage. I didn't realize then how fortunate I was, even when my dad said that my salary was more money than he had ever made in a year.

> **PN:** *Dad tells Stuart his starting salary is more than his dad ever made. This may reflect Stuart's sense that his father will not accept him.*

The first year of teaching high school was a wonderful adventure. Compared to the effort I had put in each day in college, the work didn't seem hard at all. I taught three American history classes and two English classes. In American history, I had each class divided into committees, each committee having something to do with the teaching of the course. The busiest committee was the teaching committee. Its members directed the class by means of learning games. We had a wonderful time. I worked with a fine principal, superintendent, and faculty. In teaching English, I had my students work with the nature of words, then sentences, then paragraphs, and finally essays.

But on May 13, 1966, I had a life shattering experience. The day before, my dad and I both had stayed home from work with bad colds. Dad and I talked and talked. That night I wanted to cook Dad a steak, but he said that he wasn't hungry. His lips looked blue. As he went to bed early, to my surprise, because he never went to church, he said that if I want to get married, I should go to church. The next day I went to school while Mom, also a teacher, stayed home from school to help Dad. That afternoon I had to stay late at school since it was my turn to proctor misbehaving students who had to stay after school. When I got home, I was shocked—Mom said Dad was in the hospital. I promptly drove Mom and me to the hospital. We went up to my father's room and found the door locked. A nurse came over and told us that my dad had died. He had had a breathing disease and died from heart failure. Our doctor gave my mother some strong tranquilizers to take. When we got back in my car to go home, I threw up. Mom and I were quiet with each other and comforted each other.

The next morning when I got up, the shock struck me again. Dad was gone! In the hospital, our doctor said I was now the man in the house and should take care of my mother. I took his words very seriously. My brother flew in for the funeral. He cried. My dad's mother who was still alive also came. She was gentle and kind to everyone. In a few days, I drove her home in the late afternoon, having to be prepared to teach the next morning. When I got back to the classroom, my work served as an antidote to what could have been a serious depression. I remember how comforting it was when students came up to me and said that they were sorry to hear that my dad died.

When summer came I was ready for fun. By submitting term papers, I completed three of the six courses I had taken at Green. I went to the beaches along Lake Michigan almost every day for a sun tan. I took Mom on lots of rides.

PN: *Note Stuart is ready for summer; he has a good time.*

Near the end of the summer, I got an apartment next to the movie theater on Lake City's main street. I didn't realize how cruel I was being to Mom by leaving her alone. It was a small apartment in a large grey house. My door led directly to the outdoors. I had one room for my kitchen and living room. I put my rock collection in the living room to divide it from the kitchen. I had a radio but no television.

When my second year of teaching began, I sported a mustache and a nice new blue suit to go along with the rest of a very nice wardrobe. I had a deep tan and really felt fit. Now all five of my classes were 11th-grade American history. I had all the students I had the year before in 10th-grade English. Things seemed to be going really well. I taught some of my class the way I taught American history the year before and taught a few with a contract system as suggested by my principal, a system that obliges each student to do a certain amount of work for a given grade.

I was dating a very nice woman, the gym teacher. I took her to dinner at a beautiful restaurant on Dove Lake, to a movie in River Bend, to a high school football game, and to the high school homecoming. We had good times but I found I was starting to get exhausted easily. I couldn't seem to gain any weight even though I only weighed 125 pounds.

> **PN:** *We can note that the emotional intensity involved in beginning to think about getting interpersonally and sexually involved, along with the increased responsibility that this might demand, may have increased the chances that Stuart's vulnerability to psychosis would emerge again in the form of psychotic ideas. There is some evidence that the emergence of psychosis occurs when people who are already biologically vulnerable to psychosis face increased pressures (Green, Neuchterlein, Ventura, & Mintz, 1990; Harrow et al., 1995). We still do not really know all of the biological and psychological factors involved in psychosis.*

Each day, I drove Jack, a crippled boy, to high school and back. I started saying strange things to him, such as that I believed the more money people spent, the more they would get. I also believed students and teachers were beginning to talk about me.

> **PN:** *From the standpoint of the mental health professional, one can again see strange and delusional ideas beginning to develop in Stuart.*

When a government congressman talked to my class, I said I didn't like the way he used the word Government. He implied that I was a Communist when I said that nobody should be a millionaire. I thought no one should be worth that much. Eventually I thought that the entire high school was playing a game with me. One day in November, I had classes in the morning and parent-teacher conferences in the afternoon. In the first class that morning, I showed a movie dealing with the Monroe Doctrine. The President's Cabinet looked so serious in the film, I thought the film was a joke. Since I assumed that the film was made just to confuse me, I took the film and threw it in my wastebasket. Then I left school and drove to my apartment. I thought birds were following me. The sun seemed to be shining extra bright just for me. I thought that this was all in good fun, that the school system was just playing a game with me.

When I arrived at my apartment, the telephone rang and rang but I didn't answer it. It was all the game, and I thought I would play along. I drove my Mercury Comet out to Lake Michigan and walked along the beach. It was a marvelous November day. The sun was out, the sky was blue, and the waves pounding in along the beach seemed glorious.

After having completely relaxed, I drove to my mother's house, which seemed to have a strange perfumed odor. I put on a record of music written by a famous Finnish composer. It made me cry because it reminded me of a beautiful Finnish exchange student I had taught the year before, Seka. I loved her intensely. She was brilliant. She got a perfect score on one of my American history tests, the only student to do so. I didn't expect anybody to get a perfect score on my tests. They were meant to be a real challenge. I made them up myself and gave out As to students with less than perfect scores. As the day continued, my love for Seka grew. I came to think that at the end of the game people were playing with me, I would get to marry Seka. I believed that she was staying in town at my aunt's house and that she was being kept hidden from me.

> **PN:** *Note Stuart's paranoia begins again. Perhaps this has been elicited by living on his own. He feels that others are playing a good-natured game with him. Stuart begins to become infatuated with a fantasy of a Finnish exchange student named Seka whom he had taught a year ago.*

When I was in my apartment, I played the radio constantly. I thought all the radio programs were set up as part of the game. Songs were written, love songs, just for Seka and me—songs such as "There Is a Hush All over the World." That's how it began anyway. Once I thought I saw Seka way ahead of me on the main street of Lake City, just walking out of reach. I thought that eventually we would travel around the world as international citizens, ambassadors of good will. We would travel being carried by a huge balloon.

PN: *Note Stuart's grandiosity regarding his relationship with Seka.*

One night I left my apartment and went to my mother's house, She was gone. I thought that she was with Seka. I took hundreds of slips of paper and wrote "Seka" on each one of them and put them all over the house to demonstrate how much I needed Seka. I cried and cried, I missed her so. I wrote poems dedicated to Seka, and I thought of the children we would have. She was in my thoughts every day. I continued to listen to the radio, thinking a code was being sent to me. I wrote all kinds of words for the code and came to the conclusion from what I wrote that my Dad was still alive and that he was part of the game too. I listened to Frank Sinatra sing "Shot down in April. . . ." My birthday was in April, so I thought that he was singing to me. The song went on, "I've been a prince, a pauper, a pawn and a king," and ended, "I think I'll roll up in a big ball and die." I thought that he was referring to the humor of the game. Another song that I thought referred to me was "Winchester Cathedral."

> **PN:** *One can see here and throughout this book that much (or all) of delusional materials comes from ideas, at the times jumbled up mixes of ideas, from the patient's inner life. While there are millions of potential ideas a person can have, the delusional idea is not random but comes from a limited number of themes about oneself. One usually finds delusional ideas centered about oneself and coming, at least in part, from views of what others are doing to oneself, or what one can do to others, or about one's powers, one's status, or one's state of being. Thus, delusional ideas usually are centered about oneself.*

I thought everyone was aware of me, including the people I saw downtown. When people opened their car doors, they were inviting me to get in. When they ate in restaurants, they pointed their silverware in ways that would get my attention. The lunch counter in a dime store vibrated for me.

I drew pictures of the furniture in my mother's house, a fairly good one of the piano. I drew pictures of the furniture in the August College library. I mailed one of the pictures that I drew to an exchange student whom I had from Brazil the year before. (Then when I went in a grocery store the shelves seemed empty—for some reason only for me.) I drew pictures for my grandmother's birthday present, pictures of her furniture going back to when I was a child. It was such a light drawing that she could hardly see it. But she thanked me.

For a number of days, I took long fascinating drives in my car. I drove out past orchards along Lake Michigan. I was fascinated by the design of the trees.

I thought that they were all especially constructed to be a new type of Disneyland. And all with me in mind. Once I drove quite a way north on a beautiful autumn day. A school bus went by full of kids, and I thought that they were all aware of me.

After a few weeks, I just stopped driving my car. (One day a man knocked on my door. I answered, and he had the keys to my car. He gave them to me and said I left them in the car and that somebody could have stolen it. I thanked him, but I thought no one would steal my car. People liked me too much to do that. The man must be part of the game. Besides, I thought, when the game was over, I would get the nice new Mercury Cougar parked at the Mercury-Lincoln dealership just down the street from my apartment.

PN: *Note the abruptness of Stuart's actions: He simply stopped driving his car and left the keys in car even though he enjoyed driving.*

My mother came to my apartment and I told her to go away. It was part of the game. My mother was always nice to me and laughing. I figured she knew about the game that was going on. She was wonderful. She was dating a nice guy, the janitor at her school. He was always happy too and knew about the game.

I thought my mom was having a wonderful time with the game. Besides, I had the illusion that a brilliant professor of philosophy I had at August College had been appointed as Mom's special comforter. He was a wonderful man, and I thought that he was seeing her and talking to her and just comforting her with his wisdom.

I walked everywhere, no longer using my car. There was snow on the ground by December and it was cold. I looked at bare trees, and they looked unique and beautiful to me. Everything was beautiful. Everything contained God's love. When I looked at a tree, every part of it seemed to be something to marvel at. And the tree was itself connected to everything else, including the stars and the beautiful black spaces between them. And everything was connected ultimately to God.

PN: *Again note the religious theme: The environment seemed to contain God's love; Stuart becomes more poetic. Everything seemed connected to everything. On the one hand this involves a sense of fullness. On the other hand, this involves a lack of boundaries that, at its worst, can be associated with psychosis.*

On cold, clear nights, the stars and space seemed to be filled with God's love. I wonder, wow, is this what Vincent Van Gogh was thinking of when he painted his famous "Starry Night"?

> **PN:** *One can see that at some level the patient knew he was ill and this, along with other personal material, sparked him to think about Van Gogh who also became mentally ill. One can see here that the ideas that emerged were due to a variety of factors including some knowledge of the patient about his own mental condition.*

All of my walks seemed wondrous. One night I walked on the August College campus. It was Christmas vacation, so I was the only one there. I walked into the Pine Grove, a lovely group of trees in the center of the campus. The trees cast big shadows on the thick snow in the moonlight. I came to the steps of Brown Hall where I had attended so many of my classes. I thought of just lying there and sleeping the night on the steps, but finally, I walked on. I walked past Central Park, the old town square. A few days later I wrote a poem about a ghost sailing ship anchoring above the park.

Sometimes, I would walk around town early in the morning while it was still dark out. I remember that the sound of my footsteps on the ice of the sidewalk seemed to travel down the length of the main street.

I walked several miles one winter night to meet my mother, grandmother, and aunt at my grandmother's house. They were so kind to me I was sure that they were aware of the game. Many of my high school students visited my apartment. They would just come into my living room and sit and be with me. They came week after week. They kept asking me to come back to school to teach. I knew I would be back when the game was over. But I appreciated the young men and women for paying their respects. I had sent a letter of resignation to the Superintendent, and he had accepted it. But I thought that was just part of the game. Surely they would never really drop me.

I often went to movies in the movie theater just a little ways from where I lived. I could never stay through a whole movie. My heart would beat furiously. Everybody there seemed aware of me and to be talking about me in whispers. I became convinced that a movie film trapped a part of the actor's life in the film. At my mother's home, I stopped watching westerns on television, thinking it a certain type of hell. Maybe that is what hell was—watching westerns forever and ever. One time there was a children's show on television, and I thought that the woman in charge was making fun of me. Another time, as I was watching a football game on television, the crowd stood out from the background of the playing field and seemed to be cheering for me.

I would look at the Benson catalog and think I was given the option of picking any of the women models in it for my wife. Yet they all knew full well that I would wait until the game was over and then marry Seka.

> **PN:** *Note the paranoia emerging again and the depiction of life as a game.*

The covers of magazines all began to have special meaning to me. I thought one cover had a picture of my dad.

Once I came for coffee and cookies with my mother, her boyfriend, and his friends. I thought one of the men guests was the King of Sweden and knew Seka well. People kept offering me cookies, so I finally ate a cookie. All I really wanted was coffee. I saw no reason to eat the cookies. I was only eating what was absolutely necessary.

I heard voices a lot. I heard my brother's voice. He was teasing me as he had when we were children. I knew he was in California. Yet I knew I was hearing him in my apartment. Once I even heard his voice in the public library. I became convinced that I was hearing his voice through mind-to-mind communication. I wrote all kinds of words on cards and would circle letters in the words trying to find some code that would explain how I heard my brother's voice. I would talk back to his voice, and he would respond.

The game took on huge proportions. Not only was I convinced that my home town was manipulating things, I also thought the nation as a whole was participating in fooling me.

> **PN:** *It should be notes that Stuart is becoming more delusional. He hears voices and describes events as a game. The nation as a whole seems as if it is manipulating him. From the standpoint of the mental health professional, this escalation of the "ante" can be a sign of growing psychosis.*

In Lake City, I thought adults were playing basketball in teams in the civic center for me. Nationwide, I thought the President of the United States was going to visit me, so I was very nervous in my apartment, thinking that he would soon arrive. After a few days when he didn't come, I decided that he had changed his mind.

I spent hours at my typewriter just writing and writing. I typed all sorts of things. I thought I had worked out a cure for cancer. I typed out what I thought was an explanation of intelligent life on Mars (i.e., that the inhabitants were moving deeper into the planet under the surface and exploring inner space, just as we were exploring outer space). I believed in flying saucers and thought that intelligent life from outer space was very aware of me. I thought that space ships from other stars were coming from all directions, racing toward the earth at the speed of light, and would soon arrive in Lake City. I thought that Seka was from outer space and that she had come to Geral High School just to see me. I took much pleasure in the thought that I was the only one who knew that she was from another planet. At times, I thought that she was like an angel and that she was a pulsating light, like a twinkling star, flying at night in the clear, cold, dark sky above me as I walked. I believed she was looking after me and would not let harm come to me. At the same time, I thought there was a guardian angel watching over me and that right then Jesus Christ was returning to the earth at the speed of light for his second coming.

> **PN:** *From the perspective of the mental health professional, one can see there are multiple, partly shifting, delusions. Some of these are new delusions, and others involve delusional ideas arising from concerns that Stuart has had for some time and center about delusions that he has had for some time. Stuart begins to type for hours. He fantasizes all sorts of special cures and explanations. He has fused conventional Christian religious belief on the second coming of Jesus Christ with idiosyncratic delusions.*

I thought that Sue, who went with me to Benson to student teach, understood a little of what I was going through and felt terribly sad about it. But I thought that even though she knew how I felt, she really couldn't help me. No one would listen to her. I thought when we were doing our student teaching that this cute blonde didn't understand me but liked me anyway even with the little knowledge she had of me. And by now she even knew a little bit about how much intelligent life from outer space respected me. Sensitive as she was to me, even Sue only knew a little of what I was going through.

A famous comedian, I thought, was from Mars as I had heard him once humorously tell people. Nevertheless, I was convinced that he really was from Mars and that he couldn't get people to understand all he had been through. Through mind-to-mind communication, I thought that he understood a little of my connection with the intelligent life from outer space. I assumed he felt bad, but he knew he could not help me because people would not understand.

Eventually, the game seemed to have just gone too far. I had needed to do something dramatic to stop it! The final straw was the morning when I woke up and felt the shadow of Satan was on my living room floor. Satan, I thought, was beginning to take advantage of the game.

So I left my apartment early on a cold December morning. I was going to walk through the early morning darkness to my mother's house to tell her the game had to be called off. I didn't know what was going on and that I couldn't and wouldn't take it anymore. I walked the length of the main street, past the civic center west to Kevin Avenue. Then south to my mother's house. I knocked on the door. She let me in. When I began talking to her, she didn't seem to listen. Instead she went to the telephone. I then went to the refrigerator, took some margarine out, and casually put it in her hair to try to shock her into attention. Her eyes went wild, and she ran for the door. I tried to hang on to her arm, but my oily fingers slipped and she escaped. Seconds later our next door neighbor came in screaming at me and left.

I had failed. Experiencing more confusion, I left. My mom's house was next to the high school, and students were walking down the street to school. I thought they were talking about how nice Mom and I were. Eventually, I got back to my apartment. I just sat there in utter despair. Whatever had come over Mom that she should fear me? I loved her so much. I just wanted to talk to her.

> **PN:** *Note that Stuart has become aggressive and violates boundaries between himself and others. He puts margarine in his mother's hair to get her attention. It is not clear whether he realizes it is abnormal. He regards being confused as to why his mother is afraid of him.*

I heard a knocking on my door. When I opened it, two police officers said that they had come to take me to the police station. There they led me into an office. The chief of police came in. This was my chance, I thought, to straighten things out. I told him that I couldn't take the game anymore. He heard me out, then left the room. I waited there for a while by myself. I realized that he didn't understand. Finally I left the room and walked back to my apartment. Soon, to my astonishment, the two police officers were back again. They weren't friendly this time but acted as if I had done something wrong by walking back to my apartment. They took me to the police station, took my belt away from me, and locked me in the jail. I was in near shock.

The jail was an old brick walled room, with the toilet in the open. There was no privacy. I asked a policeman why I was there and he said, "Well, Stewy, you gave the assault and now you're going to get the battery." I knew then that he thought I had assaulted my mother. I realized that must have been because I put a dab of margarine in her hair. I was terribly tired. Later my doctor came and talked to me. He was a real comfort to me. After that I settled onto the cot in my jail cell. A policeman, an older man and very kind, brought me some hot beef sandwiches with potatoes and gravy. I ate my meal and settled on the cot again and pulled the blanket over me. The walls began to buzz like bees. I felt there were thousands of bees in the wall. The buzzing went on and on. There was no relief. It was maddening. Finally, I felt my father's hand rest on my head and I felt peace. Then voices, like the roar of a crowd, came. I felt like Jesus; I was being crucified.

> **PN:** *Note that Stuart is shocked by the way other people perceive him. The walls began to buzz, like bees. He only felt relief when his father's hands rested on his head. He felt like Jesus being crucified.*

Night settled in. It was dark. I just continued to huddle under the blanket, feeling weak, laid bare and defenseless in a cruel world I no longer could understand.

Eventually, a policeman came to my cell and unlocked the door. He said that I was going to be going for a ride and that he wouldn't put handcuffs on me if I promised not to cause any trouble. He let me out. My mother and her boyfriend were there smiling at me. They both got in the front seat of the police car with the policeman while I was put in the back seat. I had no idea where we were going. I soon could see we were going east. It seemed a comfort to be out of the jail, and I felt safe with my mother there with me. Her boyfriend seemed to enjoy the situation, and I resented his sadistic attitude. We were soon out in the country headed past Zudin and Ledville toward River Bend. It was a mystery to me exactly where we were going, but for the first time, I thought, at least someone was doing something for me. We traveled through a part of River Bend with which I was unfamiliar. Finally I was taken out of the car into a beautiful new building. An attractive girl asked me to sign in. I did. It all seemed very special and, indeed, I felt privileged. Then my mother said good-bye, and I knew that I would miss her immensely.

> **PN:** *Here Stuart expresses his resentment toward his mother's boyfriend. The policeman takes him (with his mother and boyfriend) to the hospital. Stuart reports feeling that his mother's boyfriend was sadistic. Stuart's mother said good-bye. He said he would miss her.*

I was led through the building. It seemed I had come there on a secret mission. They took me into the main hall where some patients shook hands with me. I was convinced that they all had come from outer space. They had been taken away in flying saucers and now were back on their native earth for a short time in this special hotel. In fact, they had come from outer space just to see me. Soon I too would be leaving earth on a spaceship.

I was taken into the day room. There a large window allowed me to see thousands of lights of River Bend out in the night sky. It was very meaningful for me on this, my last night, to see the earth in this fashion.

After a while, I was taken down the hall to my bedroom where I met my new roommate. He talked to me in a most complicated and confusing way about which drawers were to be mine and what I must put in them. I couldn't understand his words at all. But soon I fell asleep—at peace with myself.

> **PN:** *From the standpoint of a mental health professional, it is important to note that Stuart became convinced he had a mission. This awareness of "specialness" gave Stuart a sense of peace, and he could sleep.*

When I woke up and I saw my roommate, he talked to me in such a confident, soft way that I felt surely he was looking after me. He was a bald, middle-aged, healthy looking man who must have been in his mid-50s.

> **PN:** *Note that Stuart became convinced that his roommate, a bald, middle-aged, healthy looking man in his mid-50s was looking after him. Stuart seems to turn him into a beneficent father figure.*

My breakfast was served to me in the day room. The others were going somewhere else for breakfast. So I assumed the game was back in action again. Everything around me seemed symbolic, including the covers on magazines.

After breakfast I was taken to a warm bath. Following that I was weighed. My weight was still 125. I was given some medicine. The voices I'd been hearing soon were gone. Then I was led into a room full of nurses. I finally realized that I was in a mental hospital. I told the nurses and a man who was with them that I was being persecuted because of the game and that I was suffering because of everyone else's ethnocentrism. They took notes. Soon I was brought back to the day room again. Then I was taken into a psychiatrist's office. I was utterly drained. I could hardly talk. I wearily propped my legs up on the waste basket next to his desk. The psychiatrist said he knew that I was tired but that he needed to talk to me for just a few minutes. I saw a tree through the window, about 60 feet behind him. Trees still seemed special to me. I said that there was a tree behind him. He said that there was no tree behind him. I knew he thought that I meant that there was a tree behind him in that very room. But I was too tired to explain what I had seen. It seemed that I was misunderstood no matter what I did.

Soon I was in the day room again. One of the staff workers asked me what I did. I told him that I was a teacher. He said maybe sometime I could teach him English. I couldn't understand. Did this have a special meaning, I wondered? Or was he just trying to make me feel good? I thought that maybe he was trying to say that he thought that I was all right mentally.

I walked the halls back and forth. I saw one man walking the halls with a gait that was like my father's. That gave me a bit of security. I walked slowly like him. There was also a tall, black man walking the halls. Someone told me that he was very important and from a foreign country.

I saw a distinguished looking man who, I thought, was from Finland and related to Seka. There were so many coincidences. Like the orphan I supported in Finland when I was teaching an exchange student from Finland. I still held on to the hope that I would marry Seka.

At mealtime I was taken to the dining room. I thought that there must be a unique reason why each person sat where they sat. Later, I got a haircut from a woman. It seemed significant that it was a woman who cut my hair.

> **PN:** *Note that Stuart saw significance everywhere. This over-interpretation can be a symptom of reality distortions, or even of schizophrenia.*

On Sunday, we went to a central room and heard a sermon. It seemed a privilege to hear God's word.

One day my mother met me in that central room. She was smiling and seemed real happy, but I was angry with her for going to the police and having me committed to a mental hospital. Poor Mom went through so much with me.

> **PN:** *Here Stuart admits anger toward his mother for putting him in hospital.*

Once I played volley ball in a gymnasium with some cute girls. Later, somebody took my glasses and I could hardly ping pong. I was surprised at how angry Mom became when she learned that my glasses were gone.

The days went by quickly. My roommate had me read a letter written to him. It meant nothing to me. He treated me as so important that I thought that he knew something significant was going on that I didn't understand. He showed me a court paper saying that he was going to a different hospital. I got one too. Mine said that I was going to General State Hospital. He said that they would fatten me up there. I didn't understand what he meant because I had no intention of eating any more than I usually did no matter where they sent me. My mother told me that General State Hospital was much nicer than where I was. She told me they had more facilities to help me get better quicker there.

> **PN:** *Note how Stuart interprets the switch from Sunshine Hospital to General State Hospital. He feels something important is happening. Perhaps Stuart again is finding meaning in his environment that isn't really there.*

I had been at Sunshine Hospital for two weeks, and I thought that it was pleasant—a beautiful new building with nice people. So I thought General State Hospital had to really be a nice place if it was better than Sunshine.

Soon two deputies were taking me away from Sunshine in their car. They took me to the country courthouse where it was said that I was in need of help. Two deputies were assigned to transport me to General in their car. They talked the whole way while I remained quiet in the back seat. I was dressed in my suit. The ride seemed nice, and I felt something important was happening. We went through Geral where I taught and where I yearned to be teaching right then. Soon we were at the huge General State Hospital, which is situated across the road from a university.

The deputies took me into a large, red brick building. We went into an office. A young woman asked questions and typed my answers on what looked like a form. One of the two deputies who had transported me began crying so the woman got up and walked into another room. Somebody led me into a large hall with bedrooms coming off the long hall. At the end of that hall was a large clock, and in the hall a television set. People were sitting on wooden chairs watching it.

They took me into a room with a bathtub where I was told to take my suit off. I was given a bath. After I got out of the old bathtub, I was given a robe and cloth slippers, then taken back out to the large hall. I just walked back and forth in the hall, waiting for them to take me to the main hospital. This hall, I thought, must be the waiting room for hadn't Mom told me that they had better facilities here than in Sunshine? I walked back and forth for hours. Finally, tired, I went into one of the bedrooms to lay on a bed. A staff person made me get up. I was told it was too early to lie down. As I sat in the hall, an epileptic patient walked up and gave me his autobiography to read and walked off. I thought that he treated me like one of the doctors. Eventually he came back and got his autobiography back from me. Supper came. Seated at a large table with others dressed in gowns, I ate what seemed a horrible meal. People at my table didn't talk. I couldn't tell what my drink was. Those who wore regular clothes and shoes went to the cafeteria.

After supper I got some thorazine to drink. It was bitter, and it made me very sleepy. I asked a staff worker what my diagnosis was, and he told me I was paranoid schizophrenic. That certainly surprised me. I thought that schizophrenics had multiple personalities, and I wasn't aware of having any other selves.

I sat down at a table with some men who were playing cards. One told me that he just hadn't felt right so he signed himself into the hospital. I couldn't imagine anyone deliberately signing himself into such a terrible place! That night he and I cleaned the bathroom. He convinced me that doing distasteful jobs would get me out of the hospital quicker.

The next morning we mopped and buffed the floor in the big hall, which I learned was called the day room. Then I got a physical examination by a doctor. I told him that I wanted to marry Seka. I got more thorazine to drink. It tasted just as awful as before. I talked to a visiting student nurse who, I thought, said I could be out in a few days. I was given a shave with a razor. It hurt so much I got up and left. Then I was asked to shower. I said, "Not right away." I had resisted them so they sent me to the upper floor. The upper floor was reserved for much more mentally ill patients. The day room was half the size of the one on the lower floor and it was much cruder.

A man was standing on a table. Some men were babbling on and on, and some were like me who could communicate. It was cold in the day room and, as the days continued, it didn't get any warmer. It was a severe winter, but regularly, on weekends, my mother and her boyfriend came to visit. I cried and cried when they came. I was so glad to see them. But I was so heavily drugged, I didn't say much after a few minutes.

We didn't have a cafeteria on the upper floor, just an eating room. Lots of food was put on the plate, and I ate it all down. I had a great appetite. I would appreciate meals. After meals, I would try to get a bench to lay on to sleep. I was always tired with the heavy medication. I gave one man all my stamps for writing letters because he said that he needed them urgently. I would write letters with a dull pencil. The hospital read all the letters before they would allow them to be mailed.

PN: *We can note that the traditional anti-psychotic medications (often called neuroleptics) help reduce the intensity of psychosis for most patients, and this is a crucial asset of these medications, which make them very worthwhile. In general, however, the "traditional" anti-psychotic medications also make some people drowsy and a number of people sluggish and less mentally alert, and this can be a problem for them. There are now newer "atypical" anti-psychotic medications that do not make patients as drowsy or do not make them drowsy at all. Thus, they may not induce "negative symptoms" and depressive symptoms. More time is needed to study these newer anti-psychotic medications, however, and to establish all the ways that they are better than the older neuroleptic medications and other possible ways in which they may not be better.*

In only a few days, I was led through many halls with other patients to a room where policemen took my fingerprints and photographed me. I felt like I was some kind of creature that couldn't be trusted. There were bars on all the windows, and doors were locked everywhere.

After a while, I was taken to the candy store, and that seemed a great treat. Any time away from the day room seemed a privilege.

I slept in a room with others. I had a heavy green blanket, and my most privileged time seemed when I was in bed.

Each morning we were woken up very early. Through my bedroom window, I could see the huge tower with a building on top. That wasn't used anymore. One man, an alcoholic, said that we were living under conditions that were like those in a fine hotel. I couldn't believe what the man said. He also said that he had been through several fortunes, had flown to Japan, and expected to make another fortune soon.

Eventually, I got occupational therapy in a small room off the day room. Our therapist was very cheerful, made coffee for us, and made my activity there the highlight of my day.

Every morning a psychiatrist would come through and ask us how we were doing. The conditions seemed so terrible that it seemed a cruel attempt at civility to be asked this question. I always said "I'm doing fine" even though I felt terrible.

There was one man, a pipe fitter, who said Charles Darwin said that we were in time and space. That seemed very significant to me.

Time went on, and eventually I was taken out of the building that was called a receiving hall. Everyone who came to the hospital usually was first assigned to the receiving buildings. Then, according to their cases, they were assigned to different buildings.

I was assigned to a very old building. I was put on a floor with a variety of mentally ill patients. Some had been there for years. I remember the head psychiatrist, who ran the entire hospital, passing through. A patient who had been there apparently for a number of years asked if he could be released. The psychiatrist said that he "would see." A psychiatrist's power was omnipotent in the hospital. My roommate in the old building was very kind and would be released soon. A young man, who was very nervous, told me that he had been put in for homosexuality. He was so nervous that he could hardly talk. Another patient had been dishonorably discharged by the army, and this fact crushed him because he looked on the military authorities as gods.

Soon I was put to work in a cafeteria. To get there, I had to walk through several halls of the old building. In one hall, men would rest on the floor while watching television. They looked like hopeless cases. One of the patients was the one I gave postage stamps to in the receiving hall. I couldn't believe how much his condition had worsened in a few weeks. I didn't think that he would ever get out.

In the cafeteria, I just picked up the empty trays and carried them to a central location. Some washed dishes; some of us cleaned the tables. Afterwards, we would sit around and drink coffee. It seemed that we, the workers, were the most sane, and those who remained in the day room all the time were in the most serious condition. But there were exceptions. One man who picked up trays never talked. He would just look at me. It amazed me that he was able to do a task as simple even as picking up trays.

On Sundays, we would choose to go to the hospital church. The ministers spoke to us as God's special people. I felt it was so beautiful that all of us with all of our confusion could still worship God. And again Jesus seemed very special to me as the only one who could truly understand me. The psychiatrists could theorize, but Jesus knew. Being misunderstood, I realized, was nothing new to Jesus who had been the most misunderstood man in history. Jesus seemed to be a new truth to me, a truth and a love that really did pass all understanding. Not only was Jesus the man of the hour, He was becoming more and more the center of my life. I began to understand that I could only be something with him and that nothing else really mattered.

The man back at Sunshine was right. They did fatten me up at General. I went from 125 pounds to 155 pounds. One night a church group gave us a party and there was plenty of cake. I was so filled from the meals that I didn't feel like I could eat it, but after being urged to, I did.

> **PN:** *Note that it may be important to ascertain if this is a function of the medication.*

After two months in the hospital, I was taken to the court in Gardner. I met my mother there. The hospital wanted me back for another two months, although my mother could sign me out. I pleaded with my mom that she sign me out. She did. I could go home. I was in my suit. I felt great.

I came home, and the house felt like the greatest luxury I had ever known. It felt so good to be home with Mom again.

I decided that I didn't want to go back to graduate school right away; I preferred to go back into teaching. I couldn't get back into the school I had taught in, and this grieved me. I began to apply at all the schools in my areas, but I couldn't get a job anywhere. I drove all over Michigan applying for teaching jobs. One school system with a modern junior high offered me a job teaching science and mathematics, but I wanted to teach history or English, so I kept looking.

> **PN:** *Note that Stuart begged his mother to sign him out of the hospital. She decided to do this. He came back home with Mom. He felt great, but he couldn't find a job teaching anywhere.*

Finally, a school system in a little community north of Detroit offered me a job teaching English in their modern junior high school. I signed a contract. One of their administrators tried to help me find lodging, took me out to dinner, and said he and the superintendent would have me over nights for company. Then my mother called and said a school system right near my home would offer me just what I wanted. I was allowed to break the contract I had signed.

The next day I was at the nearby school system, the Danville Schools, where I was given a position teaching reading and English in the middle school. It was a welcome relief to have a job that I could drive to right from my family home.

So I drove to school daily until strange things began happening to me. I began to think there was a force from a spaceship trying to pull my car up in the air. One day, I told a student that yes meant no. When I was teaching, I thought that my dad was alive in his coffin and that I could hear him banging it, trying to get out.

> **PN:** *From the mental health perspective, one can see that the third episode of major delusional experiences are beginning to occur for Stuart. Note that they began to occur in conjunction with his teaching. He had stopped taking his thorazine. He thought his dad was alive in his coffin and he could hear him banging it, trying to get out. Stuart may feel that he did not have his father's permission to surpass him— financially or professionally—and that teaching represented violations of his father's wishes on both fronts.*

I was becoming exhausted. My principal called me into his office and asked me if I was still taking my thorazine. I told him the truth, I wasn't. I thought that I was perfectly sane and had more energy without the medicine.

> **PN:** *From the prospective of the experienced mental health professional, one can see the dilemma posed here. Stuart's observations are that he will be more energetic without the medication. The neuroleptic medications do block neurotransmitters and also have some neuromodulatory effect in the central nervous system. However, while Stuart is accurate in his feeling that his going off medications increases his energy, he also is facing the possibility, which has occurred, that without the medication he is more likely to have delusional ideas emerge. Even when on medication, delusional ideas and psychotic experiences can emerge. At least with these medications, the chance of the emergence of psychosis is somewhat reduced.*

I drew eights on the chalkboard in front of my class. I used a thick paddle—though I shouldn't have—on my misbehaving students. One day I pulled a hair from a girl's head and put it in my mouth. She went to the principal.

> **PN:** *Note that Stuart has broken down in front of his class. By doing this (because of his own reality distortions), he has sabotaged his own capacity to teach. He has pulled hair from a female student's head and put it in his mouth in front of the class. From the mental health framework, we must ask how aware Stuart is of what he is doing and of its implications.*

The next day I arrived at school and no one was inside. I walked into the science room and, looking at a wall, thought I could see the outline of my principal's face and could see that he was angry. Soon I saw the principal walk in with two police officers. They said, "Let's go." I said, "Couldn't we talk over a cup of coffee?"

They took me down through the basement, past the furnace, and out the door up the steps. Later, I thought that they had put me in the furnace but weren't able to burn me. They took me out in front of the school and told me to go home. Students were standing in front of the school with the superintendent. I started walking toward them. Then the police put handcuffs on me and put me in the police car. They drove me to a house where I met there with the principal. Then they took me on the highway through the Fuller Forest to Fuller, the county seat. I was put in jail there. I thought that a student I knew at Green University had been in the jail just before me and that he was from another planet and he would help me. I was served some soup in the jail, and I thought that it contained the flesh from dead people. I ate it anyway, thinking that I didn't want to starve.

I wasn't at the jail long before I was taken to an enormous, old house, the Decker Sanitarium, in the small community of Decker. It didn't seem like a mental hospital at all. I asked a nurse what she would do if I raped her. It was just a warped sense of humor. Almost immediately, I was put in isolation in a small room. I had to use a container to go to the bathroom in. Day and night I could hear a female patient asking for George. I slept most of the time. I ate little. I lost a considerable amount of weight.

Eventually I was let out of isolation and was allowed to mix with the other patients in the house. I would sit there and listen to the patients talk on the building's fine porch. There was a professor from California who had a disease that would kill him. There was a salesman who was an alcoholic. There were young people. One of them played the piano most of the time. There was a tall middle-aged man who planned on marrying a wealthy blonde there.

I played ping pong, did artwork, took walks with a nurse, and had a very well-developed program working for me most of the time. My psychiatrist, a Harvard graduate, was very kind.

I got shock treatments twice a week. I would be in my pajamas and then I would lie down and I would be given a cloth to breath through to put me to sleep. The shock treatments made me feel a lot better. But I still had a few strange ideas. Like when I hit the ping pong ball, I occasionally thought that it was mysteriously directed. I didn't think that I was mentally ill enough to be in the mental hospital. I was angry that I had been taken away from teaching. I didn't think I had a chance of getting another teaching position after having been through two teaching jobs so fast.

> **PN:** *This is extremely important. His loss might be his salvation. He is angry that he has been taken away from teaching. Yet this could be his salvation as it avoids betraying his father without seeming to walk in his footsteps. Some schizophrenic patients often have this dilemma.*

My mother and her boyfriend took me home on weekends. I visited one of the middle school teachers and yelled that it was terrible that I had lost my teaching position. He and his wife just listened without comment.

After four weeks, my psychiatrist Dr. Jack said that I could leave the mental hospital if I wished, but that he would really like me to stay two weeks longer. I never considered his advice. I was eager to get out and be in the free world. My mom came up in my Buick and I drove us home. Dr. Jack did not prescribe any medicine and I felt great as a result of the shock treatments.

It felt good to be home with Mom again. But soon she was in St. Vince's Hospital in River Bend having an ulcer on her ankle treated. She had had the ulcer for many years and it had grown a thick crust on it. It limited her walking activities for she could not stand for long periods of time with it. Her doctor, Dr. Johnson, removed the crust and attempted to heal the ulcer.

I drove up to the hospital and visited Mom frequently. Her roommate was from Australia and I talked to her, thinking she knew something of me. My mental illness was already creeping back.

After Mom got out of the hospital, she took a five-week trip and visited my brother in California. She called me long distance many times. I went the mall in River Bend and bought her a beautiful vase.

There was an art show in the Lake City Civic Center. I was given a spot, and I displayed my childhood art and art I had done crudely when I was mentally ill. I had unrealistically high prices on them. I stood by my artwork proudly thinking that it was really significant. Some people I knew talked to me, but they were too kind to say anything cruel to me.

After the art show, I painted some pictures with oil colors. One was of a large pyramid, like in ancient Egypt. I thought that it was a classic and mailed it to one of the students I had had in high school. I also cut pictures out of my space books and science magazines and sent them to the high school I used to teach in. I drew pictures and sent them to the teachers and the superintendent. I sent a flying saucer book to the President of August College. He was a noted scientist, and I thought that this book would give him valuable scientific information. When I mailed the book, the envelope it was in was covered with stamps. The college president sent me a kind letter, thanking me for the book, and a free copy of a book giving the history of August College. The way people treated me so kindly with my weird actions merely bolstered my confidence in what I was doing.

I took my Buick on a trip to Ontario, Canada. I drove past a mental hospital in an Ontario city. Then I went to a motel. The owner asked me my occupation. I told him that I used to be a teacher. He said that was fine and he could give me a teacher's discount. I had trouble opening the motel door with the key and did not realize what I was doing until an irate housekeeper told me that I was trying to open someone else's door.

The next day I drove along Lake Erie. I stopped to pick up a hitchhiker, but he declined, saying he was going to a different place than I was going. I parked by a field and walked past some beautiful flowers that I thought had special significance. I stopped so fast at a hot dog stand that a mailman eating a sandwich there said that he thought I was going to hit him with my car.

I drove along a river separating the United States and Canada. I took a ferry out to an island that had Indians. I asked them if they had been investigated by a sociologist. I visited with people wherever I went. Finally, I drove home.

It wasn't long before I enrolled in a course in English novels with Dr. Borst at August College. It was a summer course, and I was just auditing it. Dr. Borst kept telling me that I should go to graduate school. A friend of mine, who I went through August College with, was now teaching a course there. I saw a girl in class named June, and I thought that she was the June I knew when I was six years old. There was a beautiful girl named Judy, and I would sit next to her and stare at her. I would scribble designs and symbols all over note cards as Dr. Borst lectured. When we were given tests, I would draw a picture and hand it in. One day my whole body shook in class and everyone noticed.

> **PN:** *Here Stuart's delusions seem to be increasing again as he approaches "forbidden territory." He enrolled in a course in English at August College. His behavior becomes stranger. He draws pictures instead of writing exams. His whole body shakes in class.*

On the Fourth of July, I drove my Buick down south to southern Alabama. I meant to drive to Florida, but I got lost. I parked the car and slept in it in the woods. I only slept a little bit, woke up, and began driving again. I drove down highways, old paved roads, even gravel roads, just as long as I drove north. I managed to get back to Lake City. It was near midnight when I approached Lake City, and there was lightning in the clouds over the city. I thought that if I didn't get back when I did, the entire city would have been destroyed in a storm.

I was back in the summer school classroom at August College. I put my pen up to my nose and pointed it toward Judy. I did all kinds of odd things. It's a wonder that Dr. Borst allowed me to stay in the classroom.

After I finished my course with Dr. Borst, I sent him letters that I thought were important. I sent vaudeville advertisements that my dad had saved. I thought Dr. Borst would be proud to have these. I sent a letter to his friend, Dr. Jones, contending that his brother hadn't died but was living at a certain address. I thought that I was right.

I sent what I thought was an invention every day to a woman's magazine. I sent little notes to mayors of different cities. One Canadian mayor wrote back that he couldn't read my writing but would answer a letter from me if he could read it. I asked one mayor why trains didn't go on the Mackinac Bridge. He wrote back that he didn't know why. I sent a letter to the editor of the local newspaper that was published. I also sent a letter to the Lake City Council suggesting that the city purchase bulletproof vests for the police. My suggestion was published in the city newspaper under the council meeting report. I sent drawings to Shady Creek, a mental hospital in River Bend. They saved them and sent them back to me.

I bought film and photographed at least 40 pictures. I took pictures of crumbling, deserted houses on Lake Michigan. I photographed some big, old trees. I photographed an old stone building that only had part of some walls and a foundation left. I thought that all of these pictures had special meaning.

I thought that the muscle men depicted in magazines were from another planet. I thought that the mountain highways were so skillfully constructed that they were made by people from outer space. I thought that there was a special place near Warm Harbor, Michigan, that went into another dimension. I thought that there was another land floating above the lower peninsula of Michigan in another dimension. I thought that there were little people living in the woods with a leader called the high scotch. I thought that one of our neighbors ate somebody. I thought that a big dune on Lake Michigan that I used to visit with a hollowed out center was an ancient space port.

> **PN:** *One can see the Stuart is describing a series of inner-life delusions and strange experiences that occur over time for him. Stuart begins to hallucinate regarding another dimension.*

I sent literature to my minister. I wrote my bank that I didn't want interest on my savings account because I thought that it was unBiblical. I gave a history professor a book about the prophesies of the Great Pyramid that my dad had kept in his library.

I thought that I would build Lake City into a great city with a nuclear powered windmill and lights that would shine one thousand miles up in the sky. I believed that my inventions would make me very wealthy and I would provide for myself and my mother.

I put Peptol Bismol and mustard on our front tree. I strung strings and tubes outdoors to communicate with outer space and to do research. In the kitchen, I put things together on the table and acted like I was piloting a ship. Dear Mom put up with all of this.

I thought that the sun had a mind, and sometimes I would go outdoors and swing my fist at it. I thought that the wind and the rain sometimes fought me. I gave magazines and books to a neighbor whose son was a scientist, with certain sentences underlined that I thought revealed scientific secrets.

I thought that my mother was an orphan in an Asian desert. I thought that she had been separated from her parents in a sand storm. I thought that my grandfather was a foreign ambassador who adopted her and brought her to the United States. I would see my mother sleep on the davenport and think of her as a poor adopted orphan girl.

I took my mother on a weekend trip to Canada in the late Fall. I drove us through Detroit and through the tunnel under the river to Canada. I was going to show her what I had seen when I went there earlier alone. I thought a flying saucer was flying over us and protecting us. Soon we were home again.

One day I put a sign in the front yard of our house on a tree, inviting high school students to come in and have coffee. The high school was near us. My mother's boyfriend tore it down.

Soon police came. I asked them if they had a search warrant. They didn't and left. I called the FBI for help. Then the police were back. I knew it was hopeless to fight. As I walked out, I saw a neighbor staring at me through the window. Soon I was riding in the police car. I said to the officers, "it is your job, but for me it was my life." They said nothing. I wasn't afraid of going to jail. Jail was easy. It was General State Hospital that I feared. I dreaded the endless hours of sitting, wanting desperately to go to bed because of the heavy medication. I hoped that I would go to Decker or Sunshine.

I was put in the Grayson County jail. I signed in. I could hear thousands of voices cheering me outside the jail. I was wearing a short sleeve shirt and shorts even though it was December. I weighed 125 pounds and hoped that I wouldn't get heavy again. I just slept or lay awake. I thought that my grandfather had become the President of the Galaxy after he died and that he had the walls of my jail cell painted the same green as the walls of the living room of his previous home to comfort me and let me know that he was watching over me. I thought he had a superior power.

On Christmas day, I was given a box of candy. I ate it all at once, thinking I might have to leave soon and leave the candy behind. On that Christmas day there was hardly anybody in the jail. People came and sang songs over the speaker system.

There was some drawing paper, and I drew a picture of a rocket blasting off. I thought that that had special significance about my freedom.

New Year's day came and I was still in jail. I had become familiar with my routine, with sleeping at night with the light on, and with eating the bland meals. Eventually, an older man was also put in my cell. We got up one morning and said good morning to each other at exactly the same time. I thought that had special significance. I called him Doc, thinking that he was a retired doctor. I thought that Doc was looking after me. He said nobody could get to us in the jail, that we were protected. After only a few days, he was gone and I was alone again.

> **PN:** *This may indicate Stuart's need for a protective father figure, something strikingly missing in his own relationship with his father.*

Soon, I was taken out of the jail and put in the sanitarium in Decker. I was delighted. Dr. Jack came to my bedroom and put his arm around me. I felt great compassion. That night I was asked what kind of a soft drink I wanted. The next day in the living room I saw all new faces except for a senile old woman who apparently lived there permanently.

Later that day, Mom came and said I was going to General State Hospital because Decker Sanitarium didn't have the necessary facilities for me. I said "what about Shady Creek in River Bend?" She said that she couldn't afford it. Her voice was full of love, and I knew that Mom would never hurt me.

I was again taken to General and given a bath and put in a robe and slippers. This time I was immediately put on the second floor. One of the men who ran the floor remembered me and put his arm around me. I was asked some questions and when asked where I was, I said in humor that I was in a university. Some of the same patients I had seen the time before were back again.

Mom and her boyfriend came every weekend to see me. I cherished their love, especially Mom's. My minister came to see me regularly. One time he said something I'll never forget, "If God be for me, who can be against me?" Those words have helped me to keep going for many years.

> **PN:** *These words of the minister seem important for Stuart's sense of well-being. From the point of view of the mental health professional, this belief may represent a positive use of religious faith to help Stuart cope with difficult times.*

My friends Bill and Linda Jardis from Indiana came and visited me regularly. I had known Bill since I was in the second grade. I got to know Linda well in visits to Indiana later. It gave me a great sense of meaning to see them. They were driving over a hundred miles each way in the winter to see me. Bill just smiled and laughed and never said anything to me about being mentally ill. He talked to me as he always did—as a sincere, good friend.

Then, too, a friend from Lake City showed up as a patient. I knew things would get better. I just had to have faith in God.

I met a 39-year-old teacher who became a good friend. We talked and walked together. We just stood around together. There wasn't much to do in the receiving hall. One day I paced so much that one of the staff workers told me to stop pacing. So I sat on my hands in a chair so that I could stand the tension. It was terribly difficult. Sometimes I cried. Once when I cried, one of the staff gave me a dust broom to push and that helped immensely.

Eventually, I got to work in the cafeteria. I wore white clothes for that position and that was a mark of distinction. I was put to washing dishes. I couldn't keep up. A nice, middle-aged man offered to take my place and let me have his, stacking trays. One of the staff asked me who had assigned me that position because I was supposed to work up to it. I said that I didn't know and I didn't in a way, because I didn't know the man's name. There was a teacher from Warm Harbor who worked there as a patient. He looked down on the other patients as beneath him.

I worked in the cafeteria three times a day, each time under a different staff worker. One staff worker said I was doing my work all wrong. She yelled at me every day. She was so grumpy I got fond of her because never once did she say that she would drop me. Later on we were allowed to take ice cream out of the freezer and I loved it. I felt very close to the group I worked with.

Eventually, I was moved to Moore Hall, a large old building that was very comfortable to live in. I even had my own bedroom. My 39-year-old teacher friend was transferred there too. We all had grounds permits, allowing us to leave the building and walk the grounds. I still worked in the cafeteria. When I wasn't working in the cafeteria, I usually slept.

A great variety of people lived at Moore Hall. Some would always be there. Some even worked on jobs in the city during the day and just stayed in the building on nights and weekends.

After I got to Moore Hall, my mother and her boyfriend came and took me home on weekends. I would go to church on Sunday morning with Mom, and it seemed a real treat to be with normal people again. The weekend would go really fast, and it seemed a letdown to go back to the hospital Sunday afternoons. One time I got back and one of the cafeteria workers hugged me and cried—he had missed me so much.

On my birthday, my mom brought a big birthday cake to share with the other workers in the cafeteria. I was 27 years old. Time marched on, it got warm out, and it seemed I would never get out of the hospital.

I got to know people that I otherwise would think strange if I hadn't been around them so long. There were two homosexuals who would dance together. One of them showed me a child's picture book with a picture of a man raking leaves in front of his home. The man said he wished he could do that in front of a house. Of course, as he realized, that would never be possible. He had reached his highest level of development at the hospital.

No matter how comfortable the hospital was, it was depressing. The bad smell of the bathrooms and the peculiar mannerisms of permanent patients always reminded you where you were. Consequently, I was delighted when after six months, June, 1969, I was released from the hospital.

> **PN:** *Note that Stuart is released from the hospital after 6 months. It is not clear where he is living then, with his mother? On his own? What about his feelings toward his mother's boyfriend?*

But I didn't get a direct discharge. I was put on convalescent status. That meant that I would have to go to the mental health center in Lake City every other week. I walked there, for I wasn't allowed to drive my car for a year.

At first I had a woman counselor. She offered me a job in mental health. She said that I wouldn't make much, but I would have my own office and I would have my picture in the newspaper. She asked me to think about it. The next time I came, she wasn't there. She had been forced to retire because of her age. I was assigned to a male counselor. Every time I saw him, I told him how I didn't think I belonged at General. It got to be a bore for both of us. I still was becoming confused now and then. I thought that the newspaper had special messages for me. Once I brought a copy to my counselor and said to him that it looked strange.

After I had gone to the mental health center for a year, General State Hospital had a review to see if I was to continue therapy. I had to write a letter and soon received one in return from General State Hospital, saying that I had gotten a direct discharge. The next time I went to therapy, I told my counselor that I didn't have to come anymore. He said that he was sorry, but he wrote General and recommended that I continue for one more year. I told him that they had released me. He didn't believe me. So I showed him the letter proving it. He was astonished. I continued going to therapy a few more times and then I quit. I was allowed to drive my Buick Skylark again.

Mom and her boyfriend had treated me wonderfully during my convalescence. They took me on rides, and we often ate out at restaurants. I don't think I could have taken it without their wonderful care.

Also, during convalescence, I applied for jobs at factories. An employment officer offered to have me live in his home and work on his farm, but I don't think I could have coped with that.

In the summer, I went to a nearby state college and took a course in the political science of Communist China. It felt great to be with other students again. In late August, I began studying for a master's degree in history at

Billing University. I thought that after I got my degree, I would teach history in a community college. The load I was taking seemed heavy, so I dropped one course. I went around with two girls and had a wonderful time.

By the time the second semester came around, I dropped out of school, deciding that there weren't any openings in community colleges for teachers of history.

After I got back from college, I applied for teaching positions all over. But I couldn't get hired. Slowly it sank in that all my college education wouldn't get me a job.

> **PN:** *One can see the dilemma here. Stuart finally realized that a college education would not get him a job. This is a fairly common dilemma one encounters when working with people who have had several episodes of severe mental illness. In this competitive society, it becomes increasingly more difficult for the mentally ill people to find employment at a high level and often difficult to find employment at even a moderately high level. This creates severe difficulty for patients who once have had high level jobs. It is a source of severe frustration for these people.*

Then I tried real estate. I was hired. But I got so nervous, I only lasted two days. I tried janitor work and found myself getting terribly nervous and throwing up. That lasted only two days. I tried working in a bank. I only lasted two days in teller training and got so nervous that I had to give it up. Mom accepted me just for being me. I continued to apply year after year for jobs in factories and stores but couldn't get hired. But Mom continued to accept me. She was just wonderful.

I began writing books. I wrote children's books. I wrote high school American history textbooks. I wrote novels. And I wrote self-help books. I wrote to the best of my ability year after year. I'm still writing.

Mom read my novels and helped me with my English, and even her boyfriend encouraged me with all my book writing. I took Mom on rides and we ate out every day. We would ride to the lake shore and visit different communities along Lake Michigan. Once a week, we went to the mall in River Bend with Mom's boyfriend, and every Sunday we would take a ride with her boyfriend. At noon on Sundays, I would broil steak or chicken for Mom, her boyfriend, and myself. On Saturday evenings, Mom and her boyfriend and me would eat pizza and watch Lawrence Welk on television.

PN: *It seems here that Stuart has resolved his feelings of resentment toward his mother and her boyfriend.*

Mom, her boyfriend, and I took a trip to California to visit my brother. When we got back, Mom's stomach swelled up. She went to the hospital. Her stomach was full of water and was drained. When she got out, her stomach swelled up again. She went back to the Lake City hospital. She was operated on. The doctor told me immediately after the operation that Mom had cancer. It was removed from her colon and pancreas but remained in her stomach and near her heart. I went home and cried. I called the prayer center at a Christian University. They prayed for Mom. The next day I learned that, with chemotherapy, Mom might live 10 years or longer. I visited her in the Lake City Hospital every day. The day she got out, I took her right to a steak restaurant. She swelled up again and went to Zimmer Hospital in River Bend a few times to have the water removed from her stomach. Then she got pills that removed the excess water.

PN: *Here Stuart's mother became ill with cancer. It is important to emphasize this major event in Stuart's life.*

By Christmas she was out of the hospital for good, and we went in a snow storm to the Jolly Inn to eat. Mom was very cheerful through it all. We went on rides every day, and we ate out again for three more years.

Everything was coming along well until Mom fell. We went to Sheltered Haven on a beautiful summer day in 1980 for breakfast. Then on the way home, Mom wanted to have lunch in a little village. She walked up the steps of the Brown restaurant very happily. Suddenly, she fell backward, and the back of her head bounced on the cement. I ran over to her. She wasn't breathing, but her eyes were wide open. I ran in the restaurant to phone an ambulance. Somebody else already had called the paramedics, and by the time I walked out of the restaurant the paramedics were already with her. She had no pulse, but suddenly she got a pulse and opened her eyes. She asked for Stuart, for me. We recovered her glasses, which had fallen into some bushes, just before an ambulance was to take her to Lake City. I drove to the Lake City hospital and waited and waited for her to arrive. I found out that the ambulance broke down in the village and another one had to come and get her. Finally, she was wheeled into the hospital emergency room. I was with her as the doctor put the stitches in her head. She talked rationally.

We walked out of the hospital together, and once again I was happy I still had my mom. But when we got home, she cried for Stuart, not me, but a little boy Stuart—a figment of her imagination. She thought he was in a house on the main street in downtown Lake City. I told her there was no house on the main street but just stores. To prove it, I drove her downtown. She was satisfied and seemed better.

The next day I took Mom to church and she began crying for little Stuart again. That was the last church service I dared take her to.

Soon a clear fluid ran from her nose. Her doctor feared it was spinal fluid so she went to St. Vince's hospital in River Bend for tests. The fluid stopped, and a brain surgeon said she was all right. But she became confused again, and the surgeon said there was nothing that could be done. She cried so much. I took her to the emergency center at the Lake City hospital for a psychiatric examination. The psychologist said that she should have a CAT scan, a three dimensional scan of her brain. She had two taken over a period of time, but nothing showed up.

We continued to go on rides, to the malls and so forth. Mom just got more and more confused. When summer came in 1981, I walked several blocks around the neighborhood with Mom every day. At the end of the summer, she couldn't walk without my assistance. Her doctor found that she had curvature of the spine from arthritis and that it was getting worse. Her confusion was getting worse too. Then she fell in the house and broke her wrist during that terrible winter of 1982. I had a tough time taking her through the snows to her doctors for chemotherapy and her blood tests in the hospital. All the time, Mom was happy as could be.

I was getting very nervous from Mom's confusion and very depressed from the blizzards we had four weekends in a row in January. I called my brother in California and he flew out in February to see me and Mom. He was fine, and it felt great to see him again. We talked for hours.

Mom's walking got to the point where I could no longer even help her walk her into restaurants. Consequently, I went to drive-in restaurants and picked up sandwiches and took Mom to her boyfriend each day to eat.

As time went on, my mother couldn't dress herself. So I dressed her. Then she couldn't control going to the bathroom, and I had to change her clothes three times a day. The situation was turning into a nightmare. I got a wheelchair and wheeled Mom to chemotherapy and the hospital for blood tests every week. For a few months, I had a nurse take care of Mom two hours every day so that I could get groceries, go to the Laundromat, and take care of other essentials. In the Fall of 1983, I put Mom in a nursing home. Also, within the last months that I took care of Mom, my social security stopped. I got a lawyer and went to a hearing in River Bend and got my social security back.

In October, 1985, Mom died. I had sold the house and bought a mobile home in a trailer park. I must have some psychological strength to have made it through all these events without a breakdown. Now I live with a schizophrenic, a man who moved in with me after his wife left him. I live successfully, taking each day one at a time. I see my girlfriend on weekends. I see a psychiatrist regularly at the county community mental health center. And I always take my medicine.

STUART'S POEMS

A PECULIAR TIME—INTRODUCTION

"A Peculiar Time" is a story, in poem form, about my stay in a state mental hospital. I want you to come with me into this hospital. The hospital is a unique, peculiar world. It is shattering to the patient who has entered it. It has to be shattering. The patient has to shake off the confusing impressions that overwhelm him/her and accept the regimen of the hospital. At first, the hospital seems to be a cold place. Because state hospitals are limited in funds, compared to most private hospitals, it is impossible for them to make a patient who has to adjust to reality feel completely comfortable. The remarkable thing is the state hospital worked. It has worked for me and for countless thousands of other patients. Not only are the workers and psychiatrists heroes for working in a difficult situation, so are the patients for striving. They are all heroes, for mental illness is the ultimate challenge. I have chosen poetry as the form to express my views of the state hospital.

> **PN:** *Stuart describes the hospital in this poem with a variety of metaphors. These metaphors may reflect Stuart's unique experience of the hospital. From the viewpoint of the mental health professional, we can start to ask here: Are Stuart's comments here the reality of a hospital? The answer obviously is that it is Stuart's experience based on the combination of the way the hospital is, Stuart's perception, and the personal forces driving him. Is this experience of the hospital unique to Stuart or is it very common or even universal among mental patients? It is both, with the poems expressing themes some of which (a) are unique to Stuart, (b) only a few experience, and (c) a great many*

have experienced, Stuart suggests that bedtime is the best time in the hospital because sleeping is a small escape from the hospital's realities.

A Peculiar Time

The hospital
was a nest.
The unsound minds
were the eggs
hatching in
the hospital's reality.
The young
chicks
were the unsound
minds

being introduced
to a new
world
of sound reality.
This reality is
startling and
the patients have
no mother hen
there.

PN: *Note Stuart's description of a hospital as a nest hatching unsound minds. The hospital is no mother hen though.*

It is a
battlefield,
the hospital is.
There is no
blood.
Only silence.
The war ended
just after the

patient entered
the hospital.
The war was
a war of minds.
Now the patient's
mind has
surrendered.

PN: *Note Stuart's description of the hospital as a battle field. Stuart feels that patient's mind has surrendered upon his admission to the hospital.*

Time stands
still.
Time is
eternal.
Time seems
painful.
Time seems
cold.
The time

is the patient's
time.
He can't
seem to do
anything with it.
But it
is always
confronting him.

PN: *Stuart emphasizes that time always confronts patients.*

Where is justice
in the hospital?
You feel like
there is no justice,
because none of
the laws make
sense.
The only thing

that makes
sense, is that
you know where
you are,
and that
doesn't seem
like justice at all.

PN: *Stuart feels that there is no justice in a hospital.*

The patients
behave like
puppy dogs.
They don't seem
to have much
initiative.
They just do
as they are
told.

And they whimper
and sulk.
But beneath
that they have
real courage.
For the hospital's
reality seems
like a whole
new universe.

PN: *A new metaphor emerges here: Stuart describes patients as puppy dogs, but he suggests that beneath they have real courage just to be there.*

The best thing
about the
hospital is
bed time.
Bed time is the
time you
escape from
your reality and
from the hospital's

reality and
reach security.
It is a security
that is so
secure, that
sometimes you
wished you
wouldn't wake up.

PN: *Stuart suggests that bedtime is the best time in the hospital because sleeping is a small escape from the hospital's realities.*

The hospital
has some good
times.
There are the
therapies.
You may make
a leather belt.
Or you may
learn to play
the drum.
Or you may
go bowling.
Any activity
you can do
is a great
release from
inner tension.

PN: *Stuart feels that activities are a good escape from tension.*

The hospital
and its grounds
seem like a
foreign country
within the United States.
There are
different rules
for those in the
hospital.
The rules are
to protect the
country surrounding
its borders.
They also protect
the patients
from themselves.

PN: *Stuart describes the hospital as a foreign country within the United States, which protects the outside country from patients and patients from themselves. From the standpoint of the mental health professional, these comments are very interesting. A boundary exists between the hospital and the outside world.*

There are times
when a patient
will lose his
temper.
When that
outburst takes place
it is both
a sad thing and
a happy thing.
A sad thing
because it is
self-defeating.
A happy thing
because it, in
its own way,
is freedom
and self-expression.

PN: *We can note that the theme of freedom and self-expression is an important theme to Stuart and a source of strength for him. Losing his temper is both a sad and a happy thing. It is sad because it is self-defeating; it is happy because it is a means of self-expression.*

The hospital
represents the meeting
of a vast array of
human minds.
It is staggering,
the variety of
minds at the
hospital.
It truly is
a miracle,
that all those
minds can
coexist together.
It makes one
wonder, if this
is possible,
why not world peace?

PN: *Stuart represents the hospital meeting of a vast array of human minds. Stuart then asks if coexistence is possible in a hospital, then why not world peace? From the standpoint of a mental health professional, this connection with the outside world is a positive sign.*

The workers
in the hospital
have their
own authority.
The patients
are always
aware
of them.
The workers
seem to have
all the
power in the
world
except for the
psychiatrists.
They seem
omnipotent.

PN: *Stuart suggests that the workers in the hospital seem to have all the power. The psychiatrist seems omnipotent.*

The hospital is
huge.
It has many
big buildings.
It has a
library,
a candy store,
a research center,
and even a
physical hospital.
It almost
seems to be
too much,
just to help
our poor
minds.

PN: *Stuart sees the hospital as too huge just to help our poor minds. This represents a unique insight into the patient's view of the hospital environment. Stuart feels small as compared to this huge hospital.*

Some of the
buildings seem
ancient.
They have drills
in which fire trucks
arrive.
But we
know the buildings
are a firetrap.
It makes us
realize
that we are
not necessarily
society's
priorities.

PN: *Note here Stuart's disillusionment with society. Stuart sees the old buildings are fire traps, realizes patients are .not society's priorities. Again Stuart seems connected to the outside world, a positive sign.*

I sit on
a wooden chair
for hours.
When I get a
chance,
I sleep on a
wooden bench.
In the morning,
we move this
heavy furniture
to scrub the
floor.
We live with
this furniture.
It seems so
durable,
almost too durable
for us in
our fragile state.

PN: *Stuart feels that the furniture seems almost too durable for the patients' fragile states. This too is a very interesting observation. It is clear that Stuart is quite sensitive and perceptive.*

There is some
kindness in the
hospital.
A worker brings
me a candy
bar from the
candy store
bought out of
his own money.
A worker
gives me a
dust broom
to push
when I am crying
to work out
my emotions.
A worker smiles
and tweaks
my big toe
when I am in bed.

PN: *Here Stuart scales down his judgment of people. He states that kindness emerges in small acts in hospital. From a mental health point of view, this too may be a very positive sign.*

A worker
tells me to
drive a cab
in Australia
when I get out.
He also
says I have
hands I can
work with.

He knows
I was a teacher.
Is my mind
now off limits
from instructing
the young?
Is my education
now polluted
by my mind?

PN: *We can observe that this short piece by Stuart, along with many others in the collections, points to how self-doubts, combined with the patients disorder and his being placed in a mental hospital, can lead to greatly increased doubts and questions about oneself. For example, Stuart feels his education has become polluted by his illness. He feels his mind is off limits. Self-doubts, such as those stressed in some of Stuart's poems, can be a source of stress for patients. Going beyond the self-doubts created by the schizophrenia illness itself, major therapists in the mental health field, such as Benzall and Kinderman (Bentall, Kinderman & Kaney, 1994; Kinderman & Bentall, 1996) have proposed that paranoid delusions are a product of attributional processes attempting to maintain a positive self-concept.*

We believe it is important for the therapist to try to help patients deal with these types of increased self-doubts and to increase patients awareness of their own assets. At times mental health workers, who are trained to study patients disabilities, focus too much on only the disabilities. We believe increased focus on patients strengths also can be a great help. As one can see, the next piece is influenced partly by Stuart's efforts to fight these self-doubts.

I see the
sunshine come into
the day room.
Even though the
furniture is Spartan
there,
the sunshine
seems so rich
and grand,

I know that
God's universe
penetrates
everywhere
and holds out
promise to everyone,
even to me,
even here,
even now.

PN: *Stuart here emphasizes the importance of hope in the recovery from mental illness. He feels that sunshine is the sign of God. It holds out promise (hope!). This, we should point out, is Stuart's slight adaptation of the traditional Biblical interpretation of the rainbow—a sign of hope.*

Even though
the patients
are of a great
variety,
there is a
wonderful bond
between us.
We are the
meek and the
humble of the
earth.

We are those
who have been
put apart for
our minds.
We need each
other and
we know it,
we all know it,
though we never
say it.

PN: *Note Stuart's religious image here—the bond between different types of patients—the meek and humble of the earth. From the perspective of the mental health professional, it is important to distinguish "spiritual emergence" from "spiritual emergency," or to put it slightly differently, "transcendent hope from denial of reality."*

While it is
considered
dangerous to
one's health to smoke,
many of us
smoke.
We feel our time
is so slow,
our time is
so hard,

that the dangers
of smoking
seem mild, indeed.
It is as if
you weren't
allowed to
smoke, you
might as well
not be.

PN: *Here Stuart feels that smoking is essential to a patient's sense of being.*

The food
is high in
calories and starch.
It is inexpensive

food but
almost everyone
eats plenty.
There is silence

in the cafeteria
as if it
is almost a
holy occasion
to be eating
together,

something Americans
generally take for
granted.
After lining up
to eat,
we don't.

> **PN:** *Stuart again uses religious metaphor. Food is cheap and high in calories, but eating is still a communal experience, a holy experience. He thus distinguishes manifest content from latent process and is able to find meaning in concrete actions and experiences. From a mental health framework, this is a very positive sign.*

In the summer
the grounds of
the hospital are lush
with growth.
It is then
that having a
grounds permit
seems priceless.
To walk those
limited grounds

out in God's nature
seems so good
that at times
one feels ecstatic,
even though
one can see cars
carrying normal
people off
in the distance.

> **PN:** *Stuart compares lush hospital grounds in summer to God's nature. He is still aware of his "apartness," seeing normal people in distance, going through normal activities.*

When I left
the receiving building
and went to
another building,
I felt something
like I did
when I graduated
from college,
but even more.
My mind

had been upscaled
to the extent that
I could be
put in a more
stable environment.
Who says there
isn't evolution?
I had evolved
myself.

> **PN:** *Stuart feels he has evolved himself when he moves from one building to another.*

When I was
locked in the
receiving building,
I had the
strange feeling
that my mind
had been put
on hold.
In other words,
I felt that

the world
wasn't sure of
me,
that it was
going to wait
and see for a while,
what I was like
before it decided
what to do
with me.

PN: *Note Stuart's awareness to see himself from the eyes of the normal world. Stuart feels he was locked up because world wasn't sure of him. They were going to wait to see what he was like before they decided what to do with him.*

When my
mother visited
me, I
knew I was
blessed.
Often she came
through terrible
snow storms to
see me.
It made me
realize I

was worth something.
I wasn't quite
sure what I
was worth.
I only knew
my loving
mother saw
something in me
that left
me amazed.

PN: *We can see that Stuart again is dealing with his own self-doubts and questions about how worthwhile he is as a person. This also points out how important and valuable it can be to have the support of an outside figure, although not all patients are able to use this type of figure effectively. Apparently, Stuart is able to use this. He indicates his mother's visits make him feel blessed.*

I worked in
the cafeteria
stacking trays.
Stacking those
trays in my
bleak environment
seemed more precious

to me than
owning my new
Buick.
The theory of
relativity doesn't
just pertain
to physics.

I'm sure Einstein
would have
a special theory
of relativity
for mental hospitals
had he
been in one.

> **PN:** *Here Stuart has an interesting theoretical thought tied to the outside world, Einstein needs a special theory of relativity for mental hospitals. At the same time, Stuart feels the need to immerse himself in day-to-day activities. He finds working in the cafeteria therapeutic.*

There were
two other teachers
with me in
the hospital.
What a paradox,
we thought,
teachers of the
mind in
a hospital because
their minds
weren't working
right.
But just as
we could train
the mind,
the hospital worked
a miracle.
In time,
it set our
minds right.

> **PN:** *Here Stuart remarks on the paradox of a teacher of the mind (himself) put in a hospital because his mind was not working right. However, the hospital worked a miracle for him and set his mind right.*

If a pet dog
walked into the
day room of the
hospital,
it would open
the hearts of the
patients to an
extent that would
seem almost
unbelievable.
The patients
are not only
starved for love,
but they so
much want
to love.
They just
don't know
how.

They wish
they did.

> **PN:** *Stuart reports that patients are starved for love. They don't know how to get love; they wish they did. From the mental health standpoint, this observation, like many other observations of Stuart, shows a good deal of awareness.*

The visiting
nurses
were very welcome.
They were
bright flowers
in the drab hospital.
They just had
to be there
to make us
feel better.
But they did
do things.
They square danced
with us rejects.
They had a Valentine's
party for us unlovable.
So we became
lovable and
we became acceptable
to ourselves.
Because they cared.

> **PN:** *Stuart sees visitor nurses as bringing bright flowers and trying to make patient feel lovable.*

At times the
workers went
out of their way for
us.
Like when they
covered the windows
with sheets and
showed movies
or when they
made eggnog
and toast
for all of us.
They had
to work
with what
the hospital offered.
They were victims
of the system
just like us.
The wonder was
the system worked.

> **PN:** *Again Stuart shows capacity to empathize with others. He suggests that hospital workers are victims of a system just like the patients. Yet the system works.*

We had to
line up for everything.
We lined
up for medicine.
We lined
up for shots.
We lined
up for meals.
We lined
up to take our showers.
The fact was
we were always
patient.
It seemed that
the total
significance
in the hospital
seemed to be, just waiting,
with the ultimate
wait
to be to get out.

PN: *For Stuart, everything in the hospital involved waiting (in lines). The ultimate wait is waiting to get out.*

Nothing in the
hospital seemed
odd
because everything was
odd.
The patients were
odd.
The treatment was
odd.
Reality was
odd.

The only thing
that wasn't
odd
was freedom.
It seemed to
be precious.
And we knew
eventually
patients did
get it.

PN: *For Stuart, nothing in the hospital seemed odd because everything was odd. Everything was odd but freedom, which was something precious that the patients finally achieved. This last observation shows a good deal of persistence and hope in Stuart.*

When my minister
visited me
we would pray.
So I had a
contact
with the outside
world,
and together,
me and the minister,
we had a
contact with God.

It was as though
God
wanted the
minister there to
remind me
he, God,
would always be
there for me.
Nothing could keep
his love
from coming to me.

PN: *Stuart feels that visits of the minister seemed to bring a contact with God. This may be an important observation.*

When I worked
in the cafeteria,
I had a
different boss for
each of the
three meals served
during the day.

This one little woman
boss would
always crab at me.
It seemed important
to me
that she thought I was
worthy of her

concern.
I knew she would
never make me

quit.
I knew, in her way,
she liked me.

PN: *Again Stuart shows a good deal of perspective. He remembers being bawled out by a supervisor at the cafeteria. Yet Stuart felt that the supervisor cared about him. This capacity to understand the other is a very positive sign from a mental health point of view.*

When I left
the receiving building
and went into
an old building,
I had my own bedroom.
The privacy was
wonderful.
The privacy meant
that I could be
an individual.
After sleeping with others

where once a
patient even jumped
up and down on my bed
with me in it,
the privacy seemed
so special I
could hardly believe it.
I knew, then,
good things come
even when you
don't expect it.

PN: *For Stuart, the patient's privacy is the most precious thing in the hospital.*

I went to singing
therapy
and I couldn't
sing well.
I went to guitar
therapy
and I could hardly
play the
guitar.
I went to occupational therapy

and was poor at
whatever I made.
But I tried.
I tried so hard
the hospital gave
me everything it had
to offer.
Effort, even for a
bewildered mind,
is not in vain.

PN: *Stuart went to various activity therapies, although he was not good at them. For Stuart, trying itself was important. This, from a mental health perspective, is a very positive sign.*

One time,
after taking a shower,
one of the workers

called me aside.
He told me
he and the other

workers
thought I didn't
belong in the hospital.
But I knew
the strange
thoughts
I had had.
I knew how
the hospital had

helped me.
I knew the workers
weren't the final
authority and I was
glad.
Maybe the help
I received was tough,
but it was good too.

> **PN:** *One worker told Stuart that he (Stuart) didn't belong in the hospital. But Stuart knew himself that he had strange thoughts. Stuart knew workers weren't the final authority and was glad that he received hospital help. This comment indicates that Stuart has considerable perspective and awareness.*

There were two
kinds of patients.
There were the ones
who would leave.
And there were
those who stayed.
Often those who
stayed had attained
a certain peace
with themselves, an
acceptance of themselves,

that those
who would leave
did not have.
This was especially
true of the retarded,
who planted flowers
when it was warm
and shoveled snow
when it was cold.
They were God's
special children.

> **PN:** *From a mental health perspective, this is a very curious comment on the part of Stuart. He distinguishes two kinds of patients, those who left and those who stayed. Stuart feels (rightly or wrongly) that often those who stayed had attained a certain peace with themselves. Does this mean that Stuart feels that patients remaining in the hospital are healthier than those who leave?*

When it was
cold out,
it wasn't very
warm in
the receiving building
either.
I had headaches

and colds.
I would hear
of the workers'
difficulties in driving
to work through
the snow.
It seemed to

me that the weather
caused everyone
to have a common
outlook toward it.

That was a
comforting unity
I thought.

> **PN:** *Stuart observed that cold weather caused difficulties, making everyone have a common outlook. This lack of difference is comforting to Stuart, something quite understandable for someone who felt so apart.*

I would read
bits of the
newspaper that
were left by the
workers on the benches
in the early morning.
I liked the
feel of the paper.
I liked how
temporary most of

the news was.
I liked the
way the
newspaper tied
me in with the
events of the
world by merely
reading parts
of it.

> **PN:** *From the viewpoint of the mental health professional, we can note that Stuart's interest in the outside world (through reading newspapers) while he is in a mental hospital is one of his assets and strengths that has been of service to him. A great many disturbed mental patients who are hospitalized turn even further inward and are not interested in newspapers or in the part of the outside world that does not apply directly to them. Stuart's ability to avoid obsessing on himself and his problems and to look at the outside world is an asset to him and a quality that many people lack when they are in the midst of severe disturbance.*

I wrote a
professor, hoping
for an assistantship
in his college
when I got out.
I expected no reply.
Did not the hospital
read the mail?
Would they not
stop the letter?

But I got a reply,
a serious, kind reply.
The professor said
all the assistantships
were taken for the
coming year.
But I felt great.
I had communicated
with an intellectual.

PN: *Stuart felt happy when he communicated from the hospital with a professor, an intellectual.*

There was one
psychiatrist who
would always shout
when he talked to
you.
But he was
different from all
the other psychiatrists
I met.

First, he took
your communication
seriously.
And second, he always
had time to
talk to you.
So what if
he did shout?

PN: *Stuart likes the psychiatrist who shouted at him. This psychiatrist was different because he took communication seriously.*

There was one
psychiatrist who came
through the receiving building
every day.
He would very
briefly talk with
some of the patients.
One day I
told him that
it seemed we all

were just being
warehoused.
I told him that
I was treated like
a dog.
But, he said,
I was not a dog.
Then I marveled.
That, indeed, did
make a difference.

PN: *Stuart felt he was being "warehoused like a dog." The psychiatrist told Stuart he was not a dog. This made him feel better, unique.*

The hospital was
old.
It had treated
countless
thousands of minds.
Each mind was
unique.
Many minds were
released.
And yet when
I was there

everything seemed
to be standing still.
I thought of the
hospital like a
huge clock that
went through
its cycle thoroughly
and effectively.
Often, this
put me in awe.

PN: *For Stuart, the hospital was like a huge clock that went through continuous cycles of caring for sick people. Yet time seemed to be standing still. This is a very interesting comment giving us glimpses into Stuart's news of time and change.*

My change in
the hospital
was so slow,
I hardly noticed
it.
I had arrived
completely confused.
After I left the
receiving building
and went to
another building,

I had the beginnings
of a sound mind.
It was like magic.
I began to feel
enthusiasm.
I began to feel
my emotions more
clearly.
I was coming
alive again.

PN: *Stuart again refers to the "change" motif. Change in the hospital came so slow, Stuart hardly noticed it. Slowly, however, Stuart realized his emotions were coming alive again.*

I met a
man in the
hospital who thought
he was a
genius
and I met a
man in the hospital
who thought
he was nothing.
Interestingly,

it was the man
who thought
he was nothing
who got better.
Perhaps absolute
humility can
be a
building block
and absolute grandeur
is harder to heal.

PN: *Stuart observed that one patient in the hospital thought he was a genius; another thought he was nothing. The "one who thought he was nothing" got better. This reveals Stuart's Christian view of self-abdication and humility: "The meek shall inherit the earth." From the vantage point of a mental health professional, there are times when this view might be adaptive and other times when it is nonadaptive.*

I met people
in the hospital
who had been

there several times.
They seemed to
have more confidence

than the
newly initiated.
They would not
be defeated even
though they had been
defeated before.
Some vowed they

would never
come back again.
What confidence.
But then,
what else
can keep you going?

> **PN:** *Stuart observes that retiring patients seemed to have more confidence than new patients. They felt they would not be defeated even though they had been before.*

There was a
young man
who was always
concerned about
God.
He would speak
about God
in a whisper.
He did not
think himself
great,

he was just
in awe in his
great concept of
God.
It kept him
going
as steady as
a rock
through all the
confusion in
the hospital.

> **PN:** *Stuart describes a young man who was comforted by his concept of God. It kept him going, "steady as a rock."*

There were the
alcoholics
in the hospital.
They were the more
stable,
more emotional
and more
cheerful of the patients.
One alcoholic
became my special
friend.

He said get married,
have children, get
a job, any job, and
take rides in your car.
In other words
he optimistically
thought what others
consider ordinary
was just great!
And it is!

> **PN:** *Stuart felt that alcoholics were more stable, more emotional, and more cheerful than the other patients.*

I went to group
therapy twice. I was
tired.
The psychologist
leading the group told
me to run around the
room. I did. Then he
said my relatives
probably
thought I let them down. I
stayed away from that group
therapy. I worked in the
cafeteria instead where
something meaningful was
being done.

PN: *Stuart did not like group therapy. He preferred working in hospital cafeteria.*

One time
when I was
walking
outside of
the buildings
I heard a scream
come from
a building
that seemed like
it came from a
torture chamber.
But I knew
it was coming
from a patient on his
own, without being hurt.
I was becoming
accustomed to
my time here,
a very peculiar time.

PN: *Stuart once heard screams from another patient. He knew that it wasn't from being hurt by others. This comment again shows remarkable perspective.*

When it rained,
I liked walking
in it.
It seemed
so real.
It was part
of God's universe.
It seemed
that little things
like rain,
meant so
much more to
me at the
hospital, that
it was the
little things
that made life
really important.

PN: *Note Stuart's concentration on little things of nature and his interpretations. Rain indicated he was part of God's universe. Stuart liked walking in it. Little things made life seem important for Stuart.*

During my last
month at the
hospital it was
a warm June.
We patients would
sit on
the porch of our
building
and just enjoy
breathing the fresh,
warm air.

We talked
little.
Our companionship
in near silence
outdoors
on beautiful days
was enough to
sustain us
well.
What more?

PN: *For Stuart, sitting outside silently in June, his last month in the hospital, made him feel less lonely. He feels nature gives patients a sense of companionship.*

Once in a while
I would go
to the library.
It was small,
but it was
never busy.
There was a
wonderful collection
of books.

But most minds
were too preoccupied
to be able
to concentrate on
books.
And me, usually
an avid reader, I
never read a book
there.

PN: *Note that Stuart is not able to read in the hospital, though he previously had been an avid reader. From a mental health perspective, we wonder if it is a loss of concentration or another factor.*

There were
some who watched
television.
Many wouldn't.
I watched little
television, though
I did enjoy the movies.
Some played
cards.
I never saw a
severely ill person

play cards.
Some kept in
little groups and
talked.
There were a few
bullies, but they
got nowhere.
No one was
indifferent.
They just might have
seemed that way.

PN: *Stuart observed that some patients watched television. Stuart did too. Also, he watched movies. Sometimes Stuart played cards. Stuart noted that no one in the hospital was indifferent though it might have seemed that way.*

We tried in
our building
to have self-government.
The workers were
promoting it.
A constitution was
written up.
In the constitution—
with a line drawn through
it by the workers—was
"The right to bear arms."
It seems especially
humorous, because on
the whole, I have
never met such mild
people as
in the hospital.
Even their handshakes
are usually
limp.

The hospital
is at first a
place one fears.
Later it
becomes a place
one accepts,
however reluctantly.
Still later, it
seems the way
things always were,
because you are
there so long.
Finally, when one
knows he will
eventually get
out, he has
a sound mind
and his mind almost
reels from the
freedom he will have.

PN: *Stuart reveals that at first he feared the hospital ,later it became a place he accepted, however reluctantly. Stuart's mind almost reels from the freedom he feels he will have upon his release. From the standpoint of the mental health professional, Stuart reveals awareness of subtle processes a patient goes through.*

After I was
in the hospital
a long time,
I was allowed
to go home on weekends
with my mother.
So I began
living in two worlds.
There was the
anticipation of leaving

and the dread of
coming back.
But after a while,
even that changes.
It seems
like coming back
to the hospital
is like coming
back
to a second home.

PN: *Note that Stuart began spending weekends at home with his mother. Initially, he anticipated leaving and dreaded returning to the hospital. Eventually the hospital began to feel like a second home.*

After I was
at the hospital
nearly six months,
I figured I
had spent more
than one out of
sixty days of my
life in the hospital.
It had, indeed,
become a part of
my life, whether
I accepted it or
not.
It was not
going to go
away. It
would be
a permanent
memory.

PN: *Note Stuart's realization that time in the hospital will become a permanent memory.*

Being in the
hospital
was not only
being forced into
a separate universe.
It also
was being accepted
into that
universe
when the old universe
didn't want you.
The universe of
the hospital accepts
you, molds you,
and makes you.
This is much
more than people
usually consider
a hospital
capable of doing.

PN: *Note Stuart's insight that being hospitalized means being forced into separate reality but also being accepted by that reality because outside the universe may not want him. This is a powerful observation, yet Stuart does not seem to be embittered by it. This indicates a great capacity for perspective.*

I went before
a staff meeting.
I was told I
was ready to leave
the hospital.
The time had come.
I was going back
to the old
universe!
I said good-bye to
my friends.
One cried.
The old universe would
accept me now.

My peculiar time
was over.
I knew I would
never see those

in the hospital
universe again.
Or would I?

PN: *This comment indicates Stuart's capacity for bonding. He knows that when he will be released from the hospital, the old universe would accept him again. He would never see these hospitalized people again, or would he?*

My peculiar time
in the universe of
the hospital is
over.
It has been over
for nineteen years.
I still have
dreams of being
in the hospital universe.
I even dream
in those dreams

that I am thinking
in a mentally
confused way.
Sometimes, I
wake up,
relieved.
But that old
universe of the
hospital saved me
and it is still saving others.

PN: *Again Stuart reveals ability to comprehend change in evidence. The hospital time was now over for Stuart, but he still dreams of being in the hospital. He wakes up relieved that he's not there, but at the same time he realizes the hospital saved him.*

MY WORLD:
THE EVENING YEARS—INTRODUCTION

The following set of poems is to show my present condition. Just as the time when I was actively mentally ill could be called the twilight years, now my world can be related to fine evenings and be called the evening years.

I get right down to the basics. I write about my God, my friends, my home, my dreams, my slow times in the afternoon, and my view of the state of the world as it concerns me. I write quite a bit about my relationship with God, because I find I have done much reflection about the ultimate in relation to my schizophrenia.

My World: The Evening Years

1. My God
My God
understands what
it's like to be
misunderstood.
Jesus was the
most misunderstood
man in history.
Only Jesus was
misunderstood
because he was
the only one
who knew what
was going on,
while I was
misunderstood
because I didn't
know what was going on.

> **PN:** *Note that Stuart again presents a curvilinear view of social adjustment. Jesus was misunderstood because he was the only one who knew what was going on. Stuart was misunderstood because he was the only one who didn't know what was going on.*

My God listens to
me when I am
very still
at night and in the
afternoon.
He listens to my
ideas
and he knows
the sense they
make even more
than I do.
He listens
to my calm
breathing and
feels good
to know
I am relaxed.

> **PN:** *Again, Stuart's religious views seem to help him. Stuart feels that God listens to him when he is very still. God wants him to be relaxed.*

I tell God
the same thing
every night,
that
I love him
with all my heart.
Some nights
I don't say anything
but I just
think the emotion
toward him.
Love is a thought and
love is an emotion.
God is love,
so I am
caught up in him.

> **PN:** *For Stuart, God is love, and Stuart is caught up in Him. This is a traditional Christian belief that seems to be slightly altered toward what may be an escapist idea—"being caught up in Him."*

My God
makes me feel
special.
He has a
plan for my
life.
It may be
just to let

others know how
I love them.
I don't know.
But he knows
the plan
and that
is all that counts.

PN: *Stuart feels that his God makes Stuart feel special. He has a special plan for Stuart's life. This seems to be a constructive use of religion. However, note Stuart's emphasis on "My God." On the one hand, this may indicate Stuart's belief in a personal God (a traditional Biblical perspective); on the other hand, this may indicate idiosyncratic solipsism.*

My God
is so mighty
that I don't
have to worry.
He not only
is watching over me,
he lets me

know that he
is watching over me
in little ways,
ways that may
seem unimportant
to anybody
but me and God.

PN: *Stuart is aware that God is watching over him in little ways.*

My God
gives me meaning.
It is not a
meaning about things
like clothes or cars.
It's not a meaning
about stature or
power.
It's the meaning

that comes from
seeing the sunshine
come out from a
cloud
and the meaning
of tasting
cold ice tea
on a warm day.

PN: *Stuart feels that God gives his (Stuart's) life meaning through little things.*

My God
makes sure that
I don't have an

inferiority complex.
He does this
by giving me plenty

of friends,
by giving me
plenty of free
time to appreciate

things,
and by giving me
the power to understand.

PN: *This is important from a mental health point of view. Stuart feels God makes sure he doesn't have an inferiority complex.*

My God
lets me be
objective,
even causes
me to be objective
by letting me
know that he
is not just my God.

He lets me know
there are as
many worlds
as there are people.
And each
person's world
is important.

PN: *God lets Stuart be objective by letting him know that he is not just Stuart's God but God for all people. Here Stuart is resolving in his mind the split between subjectivity and objectivity.*

My God
is easy on me.
He never
makes big demands.
He lets
me live life
simply

but to the
fullest.
He lets me
feel comfortable
and acceptable.
He gives me
a loved feeling.

PN: *Here God lets Stuart feel comfortable and acceptable. God gives Stuart a feeling of being loved.*

My God
shows me beauty
in the simplest
ways.
He shows me
beauty
in Penny, the cat.
He shows me

beauty
in a good meal.
And he shows me
beauty
in listening to
some favorite
music on the radio.

My God lets me
get mad at him.
When I say
I don't like
being schizophrenic,
that it isn't
fair,
he says nothing

but loves me.
His love
is so great
that it blinds
me in
the insignificance
of being a schizophrenic.

> **PN:** *From a mental health point of view, this insight is critical for Stuart. God's love is so great that it enables Stuart to accept being schizophrenic. This belief may help control the sense of secondary depression so endemic to many schizophrenia patients.*

When I ask
God where is
the justice in
my being a schizophrenic,
he answers
with more than
justice,
he answers with
the singing of birds

in the morning,
he answers with
filling me with
a good meal,
he answers me
with giving
me a good night's
sleep.

> **PN:** *This too is very important in countering secondary depression. God responds to Stuart's question of injustice in being a schizophrenic indirectly—with the singing of birds and filling Stuart with a good meal. This represents a profoundly religious perspective on Stuart's part.*

When I get
bitter because
I don't have a
job,
God gives me a
good book to read,
a visiting friend,
a good show

on television
and much more.
He gives me
all I need
without working
and never says
enough is enough.

> **PN:** *When Stuart gets bitter over not having a job, God gives him all he needs without working. This represents a continuation of a religious antidote to secondary depression in Stuart's adjustment.*

When I read
the Bible,
it tells me
more
than I need to know
about a God
who is so mighty
he created the universe,
so intelligent and so concerned,
he knows the number
of hairs on my head
and so visionary
he knew me
before he created
the universe.

PN: *The Bible tells Stuart about a God so mighty he created the universe, so intelligent and concerned he knows the number of hairs on each person's head. This approach may be very comforting to Stuart: God watches over the details in his (Stuart's) life.*

My God
is so mighty
he keeps everyone
from bothering me,
but no one
from loving me.
He thinks I can
handle what he
gives me
because he
gives me
only
what he knows
I can handle.

PN: *We can observe that the issue of religion is seen differently by different people. For a number of patients it is a source of comfort and help, and for some it can be a source of disturbance. For Stuart, it clearly provides very positive feelings of security and helps him deal with many issues. Note that God keeps people from bothering Stuart but no one from loving him. Stuart feels God only gives Stuart what he knows he can handle.*

My God
makes me
equal to anyone
I meet.
He places me
on a serving basis,
so that someday
by being last
I might maybe be
first.
But he knows
I don't care
if I'm first.
It makes no difference
in his kingdom
and that is
what matters.

PN: *Again, Stuart's religious belief seems comforting to him. God makes Stuart equal to anyone. By being last now, he will be first someday. Being first makes no difference in God's kingdom.*

My God
sent me through
the public schools,
and then through
a private college
graduating cum laude
so I could
fit into his plan.

I may not work
and I may not
see the purpose
of what he is
doing with me,
but he knows
and that is
what matters.

> **PN:** *Stuart feels that God has a purpose for Stuart even though he may not be aware of it.*

I go to church
on Sundays
in the church van
with the elderly women
to worship God.
I have made
friends with the women.
Their view of God

has expanded my view
of God.
They see him
as always reliable
through their long life time.
I like that
for me too.

> **PN:** *God is reliable throughout life. Stuart has learned that from elderly women in Church. This belief provides Stuart with a sense of continuity.*

My God
gives me a
peace that
is so great
I don't understand
it.
I don't feel
like I have

to define it
to anyone.
It is so
good in itself.
It is a pleasure
and a thrill
to have.

> **PN:** *Once again, Stuart seems comforted by his religious beliefs. God gives a patient a peace so great he doesn't understand it.*

I feel in harmony
with everything.
It is like music.
My life
just glides
smoothly along.
There seems

to be no big
conflicts.
That's because
all the big questions
are shrouded in a
mystery
covered by God's wisdom.

PN: *Stuart feels in harmony with everything. All the big questions are shrouded in a mystery covered by God's wisdom. This helps Stuart avoid many conflict-evoking questions.*

When I watch
the news at night
on television
and see all the
chaos and violence
in the world,
I become aware

of how well
God has protected
me from it all.
My life is not
full of
fantastic excitement,
but is full of fantastic peace.

PN: *God has protected Stuart from all the chaos and violence in the world. Stuart feels his life is not fantastically exciting but is fantastically peaceful.*

There is a
simplicity
in my life
that has power
in it.
It is the
power of God,

who makes
my simplicity so
firm,
it gives me
unshakable confidence,
confidence in myself
through confidence in God.

PN: *Stuart feels that God's power makes his life simple.*

My life seems
precious to me
not because I have
a lot of things,
not because I
do a lot of activities,
not because

I have a lot
of status,
but rather because
I know God
is aware of me
and concerned for me.

PN: *Stuart's life seems precious. Not because he does a lot of activities, but because he knows of God's awareness and concern for him.*

There is a
simple truth in
my life.
It is that

I am not my own.
I have a ownership
in myself only as
being part of God's

ownership.
If God owns me,
he will not

let me get lost.
With this truth
comes meaning.

> **PN:** *Stuart feels his life belongs to God rather than himself and that He will not let Stuart get lost. With this truth comes meaning for Stuart.*

When I was
first found to be
schizophrenic,
I was looking for
answers.
Then slowly,
I learned that
none of the ultimate

answers are in this world.
The answers are
in the world to come.
And in that
world my schizophrenia
will be gone
along with death.

> **PN:** *Stuart looked for answers when he first became schizophrenia patient. Slowly he learned that none of the ultimate answers are in this world but in the world to come. In that world, his schizophrenia will be gone along with death. This represents Christian emphasis on the world to come as opposed to the present world. Taken to extremes, this can result in an imbalance that can lead to self-destructive behaviors. In Stuart's case, this view seems to be beneficial.*

My God
refreshes me
from what could
be a boring world.
He gives me
interest in
literature so
that I might

see new perspectives
and have fresh
insights.
He knows a
dull mind is
a bored mind.
He activates me.

> **PN:** *God refreshes Stuart and gives him a fresh perspective on what could otherwise be a boring world. Perhaps this provides a therapeutic alternative to the overinterpretation evident in Stuart's earlier schizophrenia.*

My God
knows that I
need to feel

important.
He makes me feel
this way while

not giving me
delusions of grandeur.
He motivates me
to find meaning

in life and
therefore meaning in myself.
He makes my life
sparkle like a jewel.

> **PN:**   *God knows that Stuart needs to feel important. God motivates Stuart to find meaning. He makes Stuart's life sparkle like a jewel.*

My God
makes me realize
the highest value
is in the little things.
It is the
little things that
seem significant
when one makes himself

sensitive to them.
Like a stone in a
shoe can feel like
a rock in the negative sense,
so a little good thing
can seem like a miracle
in the positive sense.

> **PN:**   *God makes Stuart realize the highest value lies in the little things.*

My God
does not push
me toward him.
He just gently
gives me favors
that guide me
in his direction.

I find the more
I find out
about reality,
the more I
find out about God
and then, the
more I love him.

> **PN:**   *God does not put push Stuart toward Him but gently guides him. The more Stuart finds out about God, the more Stuart loves Him.*

I have a thirst
for the clearest reality
and God gives
me a quencher
to that thirst.
He gives me
a reality

beyond all other
realities.
He gives me the
reality of himself.
I can't go wrong
with this reality.
It is eternal.

> **PN:**   *God quenches Stuart's thirst for a clear reality. God's reality is eternal.*

There is justice
with my God.
He is more
than fair.
He gave me
schizophrenia.
But with my
schizophrenia he
gave me the key
to overcome it
and to understand
more than one world.
Most people never
see beyond the ordinary.
I have.

> **PN:** *From Stuart's point of view, God gives Stuart justice. God gave Stuart schizophrenia but also the keys to overcome it and, unlike most people, to understand more than one world. On the one hand, the emphasis is on more than one world—the Biblical split between "this world" and "the world to come." On the other hand, it may indicate a delusion endemic to schizophrenia. Here Stuart finds a special mission in being schizophrenic. Is this a simple rationalization or does it represent a more profound faith?*

My God gives
me plenty of pleasure.
I have the pleasure
of security with a
fixed income,
the pleasure of
being with people
with plenty of friends,
the pleasure of
having the time to
enjoy the minor details
in life that
most people don't have time for
and overlook.

> **PN:** *God gives Stuart the pleasure of security with a fixed income. This gives him pleasure to enjoy minor details in life that most people do not have time for.*

My God
is my first resource.
I don't look
at myself as a
first resource.
If I did, I would
be bored and
I would be troubled.
But by looking
away from myself,
out toward God,
I can have the
energy and the insight
to eagerly move on.

> **PN:** *God is Stuart's first resource. By looking away from himself, Stuart can have the energy and insight to move on.*

I find God
knows more variety
than I can
imagine,
coming toward myself.
Just when I
see a ho-hum day coming,
God brings in an unexpected detail,

giving the day real meaning.
It can be an
unexpected letter in the mail,
a special on television,
or a friend suddenly
dropping over.
One never knows.

> **PN:** *God brings variety. When Stuart expects a ho-hum day, God brings an unexpected detail.*

I am amazed
at the courage
I have.
It all comes
from God.
I have found
problems that seemed
too big to handle

when they were
off in the distance
easy to handle
when they got close.
That's because
God reduced them
to the right size.

> **PN:** *Stuart feels that God gives him courage.*

The past seems
rich when I see
it now.
When I see
the future it
is an unknown,
but I can relax,
because God is continually

transforming the future
into a meaningful present
and then a rich past.
Who can fathom
how he does this?
It is a continual
miracle.

> **PN:** *Note the mental health implication in this part of the poem. Stuart states that God's miracle is that he continually transforms the future into a meaningful present and then a rich past. This tends to serve as an antidote to the disconnection of present and future described by some schizophrenics.*

God judges me
with an objectivity
that is beyond
my comprehension.

He gives me
insight that is
beyond my comprehension.
He gives me the

ability to love
that is beyond
my comprehension.
And it doesn't

matter if my
comprehension is that
of a schizophrenic.

> **PN:** *God judges Stuart with an objectivity that is beyond comprehension. He gives Stuart the ability to love beyond comprehension. It doesn't matter if Stuart's comprehension is that of a schizophrenia patient.*

I make mistakes
every day.
But God sees me
with my little broom
and he is behind me
with his big broom
cleaning up everywhere

I attempt to go.
He loves my
attempts
and he treasures
my aspirations as
I go on my way.

> **PN:** *Stuart feels God provides a buffer for him. God is behind Stuart's little broom with a big broom cleaning up his mistakes.*

If God is concerned
about the little animals,
how much more
interested he is
in me.
And if schizophrenia
is interesting,

how much more
interested he must
be in how
I will turn out.
It is exciting
just thinking
of his interest.

> **PN:** *God is interested in Stuart, in his schizophrenia, and in his outcome. This personalizes Stuart's disease in a constructive fashion.*

I feel interest
in just about everything.
It is finding
the unusual
in the small
and insignificant
that is the most

interesting of all.
When that happens,
when no stone
is left unturned
to find the interesting,
I am sure God
smiles.

> **PN:** *Stuart has a curious description of God here. God smiles when Stuart leaves no stone unturned to find the interesting. Stuart seems to be saying God wants him to first be creative.*

2. My Friends

I live with
Bob,
a schizophrenic.
Bob and his cat,
Penny,
have lived with me
for over three years.
Bob's wife left
him more than four years ago.
Bob is quiet, kind, intelligent,
and has a quick sense of humor.
Bob sees things
the way I do.
We are both
47 years old
and went to school together.

> **PN:** *Stuart describes his living arrangements. Stuart lives with a "schizophrenic," Bob, and his cat, Penny. Bob is same age as Stuart; they both are 47. Bob is quiet, kind, intelligent, and sees things the same way as Stuart.*

Jack is twenty-seven years
old and a schizophrenic.
He is short like me
and dates Judy, another schizophrenic.
Often, Jack and Judy
visit my trailer.
Jack lives near Lake Michigan
twenty-five miles
north of me.
He drives a beautiful
restored 1967 Buick Riviera
to my place.
He, Judy and I
usually all go out
for coffee
when they come.

> **PN:** *Stuart is friends with Jack, a younger (27-year-old) schizophrenic, who dates Judy. Stuart often goes out with Jack and Judy. It is important that Stuart has social contacts.*

Bill is thirty-three years old
and is manic depressive
and schizophrenic.
When we get together
at my place,
we play backgammon,
a game that has been
played for thousands of
years in the Middle East.
Bill has a snake.
He raises mice to
feed the snake.
He calls me
twice a day.
He is very active.

> **PN:** *Stuart is friends with Billy, a 33-year-old manic depressive with a pet snake. They play backgammon together. We can note that in our clinical experience we have observed that a number of former patients, after a few hospitalizations, begin to turn to other former mental patients for friendship and companionship. In one sense, many of them*

*feel more comfortable associating with former mental patients and feel
more accepted by them.*

Steve studied
in medical school
for a year to be a doctor.
He is schizophrenic and
    manic depressive.
He is very religious.
Presently, he is back
in school
studying for another
hospital occupation.
He is bright
and serious.
He drives a real old car
for he has
very little money.

PN: *Stuart is friends with Steve, a former medical student, who is
schizophrenic and manic depressive. Steve is back in school now studying for another hospital occupation. He drives a real old car and has
little money.*

Mary is my girlfriend.
Mary is manic depressive.
She is forty years old,
divorced, and has
three children.
She lives in a large,
new, mobile home.
We have wonderful dates.
We go on picnics.
We go out for coffee.
We go to Lake Michigan.
We watch videos
and we drink wine together.
I phone her
twice a day.
She's wonderful.

PN: *Mary is Stuart's girlfriend. She is a 40-year-old divorcee with
three children. Stuart and his girlfriend go on wonderful dates together including picnics. He phones her twice a day. Regularity is
probably very important for Stuart.*

Sue is a combination
schizophrenic-manic depressive.
She is a pen pal.
She got through her
second year
in medical school before
she became ill.
She graduated *magna cum laude*
from an Ivy League college.
She has a brother and
sister who are psychiatrists
and another sister
who is a nurse.
She writes wonderful poetry
and is a fine
friend.

PN: *Stuart is a pen pal with Sue, a combination of schizophrenic and
manic depressive. She was an Ivy League student who got through her
second year of medical school before she got sick. She writes poetry
and is a fine friend.*

Nancy is a friend
I made through having
day treatment in
the home she lived in.
She is very sick
as a schizophrenic.
She thinks she
hears the voices of
dead people,
who she says
are on the other side.
She is so good
and so confused.
I will always
be her good friend.

PN: *Stuart is friends with Nancy. She is "very sick as a schizophrenic"
(Stuart's wording). She thinks she hears voices of dead people. Stuart
states that he always will be her friend. This is important for Stuart.
He is instrumental in helping someone sicker than him.*

Charles is a
friend I met
in day treatment.
He would often
forget what he was talking about.
He is schizophrenic.
I consider him
my friend.
I don't know
if he considers me
his friend.
I think he is paranoid.
He can be violent.
One day
he hit his dad on the head
with a pop bottle.

PN: *Stuart is friends with Charles, a paranoid schizophrenic with
memory losses, who could be violent. One day he hit his dad on the
head with a pop bottle. We can note that the great majority of schizophrenia patients are not violent. They are not forward enough, and/or
active enough, or willing to take the sufficient initiative to push or ad-
vance their own causes. There are, however, rare, select, violent schizophrenia patients who are potentially very violent and who can engage
in behavior dangerous to society. The great majority of schizophrenia
patients, however, are not violent.*

Dave and Cindy
live in Indiana
and are among my
best friends.
When I first got
out of the hospital
and when I was permitted
to drive again,
I visited them every month.
Now I see this
married couple
a few times a year.
They accept me as I am.
I first knew Dave
when I was
a child.

PN: *Stuart is friends with Dave and Cindy who live in Indiana and are among his best friends. He sees them a few times a year. He knew Dave as a child. This is important as it provides Stuart with some life-span continuity.*

My brother
has been good to
me all these years.
He is a school psychologist
so he understands me
in many ways.
He writes to me
regularly from
his home in California.
He lets me know
that he cares.
When we were young
we had sibling rivalry.
All that is gone now,
and what remains
is a good, old friendship.

PN: *Stuart's brother is a school psychologist in California. He writes Stuart regularly to let Stuart know that he cares. The sibling rivalry from childhood is gone. What is left is friendship. This relationship too seems to give Stuart life-span support.*

My church friend
Luke
goes out for coffee
with me once
a week.
We talk about
God.
We talk about
justice.
We talk about
growing older.
We talk about
heaven.
We have found
a deep meaning
in our friendship.

PN: *Stuart has a church friend Luke. They go out for coffee once a week. They talk about justice, growing older, heaven. They find a deep meaning in their friendship. Note that Stuart has some friends who have not been mentally ill as well. This provides a good balance for Stuart.*

Dr. Carl
has been my friend
for over five years.
I used to talk
to his psychology classes
at August College
about schizophrenia.
(I graduated from
August College.)
Now I talk
with Dr. Carl mainly about
the professors I had
and who he worked
with.
He gives
a good balance
to my life.

PN: *Stuart is friends with Dr. Carl, a psychologist at August College. Stuart used to talk to Carl's psychology classes about schizophrenia. Now they talk about professors who they both worked with. Dr. Carl gives a good balance to Stuart's life.*

My aunt,
here in Lake City,
has me over
now and then
for a dinner
and to talk over old
times.
She is in good
health.
She married late
in life,
and now enjoys
the company of her husband
greatly.
She gives me
inspiration
that the old life
can be a
good life.

PN: *Stuart's aunt has him over for dinner. She married late in life. She gives Stuart inspiration that the "old life can be a good life."*

My uncle in Wisconsin
is an artist
with oil paints,
a violinist
a violin teacher,
and a potter,
and has performed
in plays on local television.
He is very talented
and very kind.
We write many letters
to each other.
We seem to
have grown even closer
as we both get older.

PN: *Stuart's uncle is in Wisconsin. He is an artist with oil paints. He is a violin teacher and potter. Stuart and he correspond and have gotten close as they have gotten older. Note have Stuart's friendships are balanced between people who have and haven't experienced a mental illness.*

My two nieces and one nephew
live in California.
I love them dearly.
At first both
nieces were going
to study to be
psychologists.
Now one is.
They love me.
They accept me.
I had to laugh, when
in one letter my
young nephew wrote
me asking if "I
ever got down."

PN: *Stuart has two nieces and one nephew in California. They love him and accept him. Stuart's nephew asks Stuart if he ever got down, which made Stuart laugh. This is, in many ways, a remarkable passage. Stuart shows awareness that his situation may cause him to get depressed and that this is normal. Stuart shows real perspective here.*

Craig is a schizophrenic.
We became friends
in group therapy.
We have worked
in perfect harmony
on this book
for four years now.
We have laughed
over a beer,
talked together before
a psychology class
at August College
and in general
formed a very
constructive friendship.

PN: *Stuart is friends with Craig, the co-author of the book. Craig is also a schizophrenia patient. They met in group therapy. They work together harmoniously and have formed a constructive friendship.*

3. My Home
I love my
mobile home.
It is easy to
take care of.
And that is good,
because, every effort
with my schizophrenia,
seems difficult
to initiate.
I wash the windows,
for instance,
every two years.
It would seem
too much to do
every year.

PN: *Stuart loves his mobile home because it doesn't require much effort to maintain. Too much effort is overwhelming for Stuart. Stuart has learned to pace himself and to budget his energy.*

Maintaining
a home
is one of getting the
right people to do
the right thing.
I always need
someone to shovel
the snow off the roof
if it gets too deep
and someone to
coat my roof so
it won't leak.
The rest is up
to me.
I like the
challenge of
taking care of myself.

PN: *Stuart knows how to get help to do the things that he can not do. The rest is up to Stuart. He likes the challenge of taking care of himself.*

Most of my furniture
comes from the
house my parents lived
in.
There is the desk
my dad gave my
mother for their
wedding anniversary.
There is the vase
passed down from
my grandfather, to my
mother, to me.
The vase looks very
expensive.
It has an oriental look.
I treasure
these things of the past.

PN: *Stuart treasures furniture from his parents' house because it represents his past.*

It gets mighty
hot in my mobile home
when it is just in the
upper 70s outdoors.
But I can't turn
my central air conditioning
on until the weather
remains warm day after day,
because the air conditioner
blows the pilot light
out in my furnace
and my furnace is
very hard to start
once the flame
is out.

When the trains go by
on the nearby railroad tracks,
my home shakes,
and when big old automobiles
rumble by,
the dishes clatter in
the cupboard.
It makes me
realize, a mobile home
is not real solid,
but this also
makes me think
life itself is
just transitory.

4. My Dreams
I dream many nights
of my mother.
She is confused
like she was in
her last years.
And I am taking care
of her,
as I was in
her last years.
These dreams come
again and again.
And though
my mother is confused
in them,
I treasure them,
because she is there.

PN: *Stuart dreams many nights of his mother. Her images are confused in his dreams, but Stuart treasures them because his mother is
there.*

I have fond memories
of my dad.
But unfortunately
my dad was
also an alcoholic.
And often
he would shout.
Sometimes, I still

dream he is drunk
and shouting
and upsetting the peace
in our home.
It is sad
that this memory
still lingers in my dreams.

PN: *Stuart says he has fond memories of his father. But he also
acknowledges bad memories because his father was an alcoholic. He
would shout and disrupt the house. Stuart feels sad that this memory
lingers on in his dreams. Yet it may be healthy for Stuart to face his
ambivalent feelings.*

I have wonderful dreams
where I am driving my car,
taking my mother
on a trip
in northern Michigan.
The dreams
are based on
reality,
for I often did
take my mother
through northern Michigan
in my car.
I no longer
have a car.

I have wonderful dreams
where I am going
on fantastic rides,
like the rides
you go on in
Disneyland,
but even more
fantastic.

The details are all
there,
but I can't
remember the details
when I'm awake.
I just remember
my thrills
from the rides.

Often I dream
I am drawing
many inventions
down on paper
with a pen.
I dream I am dreaming
this
and I try to remind
myself to remember
these inventions
when I wake up,
because they
will make me
rich and famous.

I dream
I am a great artist.
The art varies
from painting great
paintings with oils,
to drawing interesting
cartoons.
I wanted to be
an artist when
I was a child
and I think
this desire is still
working its way
out in my dreams.

I dream
I am traveling
with my parents
through the Arctic north.
It is not cold,
just beautiful.
We drive on
paved highways in
northern Canada
where there are no

highways.
We fly to northern islands
and ultimately
to modern cities
in Siberia Russia.
This dream
has repeated
itself.

I dream my
entire family
is together.
My brother and I
are living with
our parents again.
It seems
like even after
all these years,
I subconsciously
miss the security
of being a child
with my parents
even though
I am doing well
on my own.

PN: *Stuart dreams of his entire family living together. He and his brother are living with his parents. He misses the security of being a child with his parents, even though he is doing well on his own. From a mental health perspective, this is quite honest and normal.*

5. My Slow Times
The afternoons
are my slow times.
It is a time
when Bob sits back
and drinks a beer,
when I have
my ice tea
and we listen
to music on the
radio.

We usually
talk little
just enjoying the peace
in the room.

Sometimes
Bob and I
will let his cat, Penny,
outdoors
during the slow times.
We will follow

her as she walks
around the trailer.
We will watch
her eat grass,
and if she
strays, we get
the broom.
We don't
know why
she is so scared
of the broom.

After I have
had my fill of
ice tea

during the slow time,
I go off
to the living room
and lay down on the couch.
The afghan goes
over me
and soon I am asleep.
I wake up about 2:30
in the afternoon.
In thirty minutes
Bob goes to sleep
and I am left
sitting in my chair
listening to the music
on the radio.

PN: *Note the regularity in Stuart's life. After drinking iced tea, Stuart will lay down on the couch. He wakes up at 2:30 in the afternoon. He listens to the radio and Bob goes to sleep.*

6. The State of the World
The world
seems a cold, barren place
filled with pollution,
overpopulated,
always having wars
or the rumors
of wars

and lacking in
sufficient love.
The world
is suffering.
But that doesn't
mean I must suffer.
I can have
my own world.

PN: *Stuart feels that even though the world is suffering, he can have his own world. Stuart shows awareness of the outside world but realizes he also has a personal life.*

Medical care
is insufficient
for millions of people
in the United States
even though we are
the richest of lands.
It seems if
you are poor

in America,
you are forgotten.
I know many
of my schizophrenic brothers
and sisters
are living on
the streets in cities
without medical care.

PN: *Note again Stuart's awareness of the outside world. Stuart feels Medicare is insufficient for millions of people in the United States, in-*

cluding his schizophrenic brothers and sisters who are living on the streets without medical care.

I read somewhere,
that as a schizophrenic
I have a lower
status
than a criminal.
This country,
the land of the free,
has put more
stigma on me
and others like me
than we can handle,
so I just forget
the stigma
and go on living.

PN: *As a schizophrenic, Stuart feels he has a lower status than a criminal. Stuart feels that this stigma is more than he can handle. He just forgets the stigma and goes on living.*

I remember
in the high school
I taught in,
they had a
play that
had a paranoid schizophrenic
on the escape.
This was supposed
to be a terrible thing.
Little did
I know then,
that a year later
I, one of their teachers,
would be diagnosed as paranoid
   schizophrenic.
And the state of the world
hasn't changed its thoughts
about schizophrenics
since then.

What if Paul
in the Bible
was a schizophrenic
when he was blinded
and heard Jesus?
Would it make
any difference?
What is reality
anyway?
If we share
our reality with others,
is it no less real
if we are a schizophrenic
or not?

PN: *We can observe that here again Stuart is expressing his doubts about himself and asking whether the views, thoughts, ideas, and dreams of a former or current schizophrenia patient are as important as, as real as, and as worthwhile as that of a person who does not have a schizophrenia disorder. It is hard not to be moved by Stuart's plea to regard him as someone with worthwhile ideas, who is a worthwhile person. Stuart expresses this thought in New Testament terms: What if Paul in the New Testament were schizophrenic when he was blinded and heard Jesus? Would it make any difference? Is our shared reality less real if we are schizophrenic?*

SUMMARY OF STUART

PN: *Stuart's history can be seen from a variety of perspectives. One approach is to view Stuart as a person who because of genetic and/or other reasons is vulnerable, under stress, to schizophrenia. Looked at in this way, his initial psychotic break may be seen as occurring in a vulnerable person who is subjected to increased tension, stress, and conflict from (a) being away from his home and in an unfamiliar setting, which makes him feel insecure; (b) underlying conflict and concern that his attending graduate school has increased the financial strain on his parents; (c) undertaking graduate work for the first time, with some underlying concern that the work may be difficult for him; (d) some initial physical illness in graduate school; and (e) some early concern about the "overcrowding" among students. In addition to the stress created by all of these factors, and especially by the insecurity associated with living in a new and unfamiliar setting, there also may be increased conflict and stress that arise, in part, out of a conflict with his father regarding Stuart's concern that his father may not want Stuart to surpass him. The teaching profession may evoke this sense of disloyalty for Stuart, heightening stress and, in conjunction with other factors that we do not completely understand, facilitating a psychotic break. When Stuart finally succeeds in destroying his teaching career, the acute phase of his psychosis seems to lift. This view must be tempered by our observation that many young adults move into new and unfamiliar settings with increased insecurity, that many sons have conflicts with their fathers, and that very few of these people develop schizophrenia. So it is likely that the key factor is Stuart's initial vulnerability to schizophrenia, which was triggered by a constellation of*

89

stress-increasing factors, among them being his perceived conflict with his father.

Throughout his sickness, Stuart is helped by a number of constructive forces. First, Stuart stays in contact with the outside world. This is important because it keeps him from being isolated. Second, Stuart possesses the ability to express himself in poetic metaphor. If used correctly, his greater cognitive flexibility may help bond Stuart with the outside world. Third, Stuart has a deeply religious orientation. For some people with severe mental illness this can be helpful, whereas for others it is not an automatic benefit. As can be seen throughout this book, for Stuart it is extremely helpful. It enables him to see life from a variety of perspectives, to accept his condition without losing hope, to have a feeling of "belonging" and of being associated with something of greater importance, and to maintain his courage.

CRAIG'S STORY

It is 1978, my senior year at Lake City High School in Lake City, Michigan. My two favorite subjects are art and carpentry. I am a quiet student who sticks only to a few close friends, ones I grew up with in my neighborhood. My friends and I would take turns playing poker in our parents' homes on weekends. We would have beer and munchies, and once in a while we would produce a smoke-filled poker table atmosphere with our favorite cigars. Another pastime of ours was to cruise the beach in the summer to see beautiful girls and fast cars while playing our favorite rock and roll tapes. We all had nicknames for one another. Mine was The Flag; Dan's was The Man, Tim's was The Boy, Scott's was Quaker Oats, Matt's was Dip, and Gerry was Big Guy.

We would all pass the word that a game was in the making for after school with another neighborhood. It would be football, basketball, or baseball, depending on the season. My friends all seemed like brothers to me. We would see each other through the good, the bad, and the ugly times.

My friends and I did all kinds of sports. We helped each other out and always supported each other as we ventured into a new sport. While living on the lake, my folks bought a boat. Soon my family and friends were learning to water ski. During the winter, down hill skiing and ice skating took up our time. We bowled, played handball, racquetball, golf, tennis, and volleyball. Golfing was a big mistake for me. I had the tendency to hit the ball a couple fairways over. One time I managed to lose a ball on every fairway. All in all we had a lot of fun together.

My senior year during spring break Matt and I took off for Florida in my Opal GT for some relaxation in the sun. We drove straight through, only stopping for food and gas. I made the error of not using any suntan lotion my first day out in the sun. I ended up paying for it the next day with a bad sunburn. The only relief I found was to pour vinegar all over my body. After that, my attire consisted of a long sleeve shirt, pants, and a hat for the rest of the vacation. We also had friends staying 10 miles away. One day, they all wanted to play golf. I volunteered to keep score because I didn't want to kill anyone with my golf technique. On the way back, I peeled my skin off like a snake. Matt was mad at me because I'd let the wind blow my dead skin all over the car.

Holidays were a time when the family was all together. My mother is the one who recorded all the holiday activities with her camera. There was always more than enough food for everyone. After dinner we'd get together for a board game. Weather permitting, the adults would gather on the deck to talk, while the kids played volleyball or threw the Frisbee around. I treasure the moments we are together as a family.

During one winter break, my parents took me and Alex to Madrid, Spain, where my brother, Roger, had been studying Spanish. We saw the national art museum there. Everything was old. There were a lot of masters in artwork there. We visited Seville, Marbella, Granada, and Barcelona. Roger and his girlfriend, who had been studying in France, joined us in Barcelona. In Nice, France, my Uncle Don and a friend joined us. That afternoon we went on an excursion to Monte Carlo. We then proceeded into Italy. We visited Milan, Venice, Florence, and Rome. That vacation is one I'll never forget.

My Opal GT sports car was fun to drive. I liked the way it was so close to the ground, its 4-speed shift, and its red-orange color. I liked to drive up in the hills by Lake Michigan and through the woods.

The last thing I would see on television at night was the Johnny Carson Show, a talk show I liked very much. I also like to watch Phil Donahue.

Speaking of brothers, I have two, Alex and Roger. They are very loyal. Alex is my younger brother. He was a year behind me in school. I always respected him because of his ability to talk his way in and out of places. When he talked his way out, I thought he had no fear, but many times his mouth got him in more trouble that he could handle alone.

Roger was the trailblazer for the two of us. He would give us ideas about how to do things, tips on what to look out for, and how to get around problems.

My mother protected her children. She would do her best for each of us, but at times her style embarrassed me. My father is strong, alert, and wise.

> **PN:** *This is important from a mental health point of view. Craig is describing his life in high school, his friends, and his family. He had close male friends. He was close to his brothers. His older brother, Roger, was a trailblazer. His younger brother, Alex, had the ability to talk his way in and out of situations. His mother was protective but sometimes embarrassing. His father was strong, alert, and wise.*

During the second semester of my senior year, I had only a three-hour carpentry course at South Side High School, so in the afternoon I took a job at the Pizzeria as a cook.

One day at the pizzeria, when I started doing the cooking and the prep work, Pat, Kelly, and the boss started talking around in circles. It seemed as though the devil was taking over their bodies when they talked to me. Kelly started talking on the phone, and it seemed he was using a voice other than his own. That confused me. I was even more confused when he told me that I didn't have to work for the rest of the day.

I drove home and found no one there. I tried to sleep on the couch, but I couldn't. I got up and went to my car. I started it up and drove to my high school. I met Scott, a friend, there and tried to tell him what was bothering me, but he was between classes and didn't have much time to talk. I went to the school library where I found Bill. But he wasn't much help either. Then I walked over to the school office where I decided to call the police and tell them of my problem of hearing strange voices. I asked if the Police Chief would come and listen to what I had to say.

> **PN:** *This too is interesting from the vantage point of the mental health professional. Note that Craig was aware enough to seek help. During the second semester of his senior year, Craig became delusional while working at a pizzeria. He heard the devil talking over the bodies of several of his colleagues. Again Craig was aware enough to go home and call the police.*

He did. He picked me up at school, drove me around, and listened to me. Finally, he had me drive my car to the police station where I talked with another police officer. The police officer called my parents. Soon the four of us were in a room. My father seemed to understand me. My mother and the police officer were talking with me, but it seemed my father was playing with them with his thoughts. My father drove me home, while my mother picked up some hamburgers for dinner.

> **PN:** *We can note that there is not one single psychotic experience that is uniform across the disorder. Rather, it differs somewhat for different people. This account is still important, however, as it shows many features that are in common among sufferers of the disorder. Among them is that at the time of the initiation of the psychotic experience, the patient often is only partly aware of how strange he/she looks to others. In effect, many have lost the ability to monitor their own conditions effectively (Harrow et al., 1989; Port et al., in press).*

At home, my brother Alex and our pets appeared different, as though my father was using them with his brain. My father could take over people's minds and bodies with his own brain waves. My father and I would watch television together and communicate without saying a word. My father's friends from work had a club of people who practiced brainwashing different people. They wanted to practice on me. They took over the entire household except for me and my father. My father and I would think of different people or objects. We did this to block our minds so they couldn't capture our minds or bodies. They gave up the next day.

> **PN:** *Consider Craig's first psychotic break. He finds his father seemed to understand him. His mother and the police officer were talking with him, but his father was playing with them with his thoughts. Craig gives his father special powers—as if he were the director of the entire script. Craig feels his father could take over people's minds and bodies with his own brain waves. Craig reports that he and his father would think of different people and objects so they "couldn't capture our minds or bodies." It is possible that Craig is describing hallucinations as a defense against being influenced. If one thinks of a sinister figure, one controls it by making things conscious. One takes away the other's power.*

My parents took me to the Lake City Hospital to find out what was happening to me. At the hospital we met my family doctor and a couple of other people, none of whom could figure out what was happening to me. They asked questions, took my blood pressure, and took blood samples. I tried to leave that night. I was urged on from a song by *ABBA*, but two big guys in white coats took me back to my room. The next morning when I was served my breakfast, I tasted and smelled my food a little before I ate it all.

PN: *We would like to emphasize Craig being urged on by a song from a rock group, ABBA, but two "big guys" took him back to his room. He tasted and smelled food before eating it all.*

I found out that my father was hiding me out in the hospital. There was another case like mine. That same day a girl was being hidden in another side of the hospital. Some of her father's friends were trying to get me out, but my father was mixed up with the KKK. The KKK had a big meeting that night at the hospital. My father gave half of his knowledge so that I could call him back from his KKK meeting at any time. He also gave me special sight so that I could watch the meeting without being noticed.

On the other side of the hospital, the father of the girl who was being hidden was mixed up with the Nazis and the Mafia. Both of our fathers wanted out, but the organizations wanted me and the girl. The Nazis and the Mafia had found the girl at the opposite side of the hospital. They were using her to find me. They wanted to use us to rule the world. She had the power from her father to transmit the images that I saw about where I was being hidden. When I looked around the room, they would pick up a silhouette image of my father sitting in an easy chair.

PN: *We note here that this material shows how, with one's delusions and with one's altered sense of reality, one can be living in a subjective world that in one way is quite different from the real world and in another way contains parts that are consonant with the real world. For example, here Craig knew he was in a hospital-like setting, knew who some of the doctors were, etc. At the same time, however, as can be seen by the account, other aspects of his world were grossly delusional. Consider Craig's delusion that a girl's father's friends were trying to get Craig out of the hospital but that he himself was mixed up with the KKK. Craig feels that his father gave him "half of his knowledge" so that Craig could call his father back from the KKK meeting at any time. Father gave Craig "special sight" so that he could watch the meeting without being noticed. Craig is certain that the father of the girl was mixed up with the Nazis and that the "Mafia girl" received power from Craig's father. Craig suggests an idea of parallel realities. He claims that the Mafia and the Nazis found a silhouette image of his father sitting in an easy chair. In this sense, Craig's material is an illustration of how most psychotic patients are living in the real world and partly in their own delusional world, rather than being totally delusional in all aspects all day long.*

They began searching the hospital by floors. Daylight started showing through the window blind. So that postponed the search for me. My mother was always trying to expose the way my father and I could communicate with each other.

My older brother's girlfriend was able to communicate to my father with powers she inherited. She worked with my two brothers in trying to get me out of the hospital and to a safe place. Alex was an old patient a couple of rooms down from me. Roger was a doctor who would come in and take my blood pressure.

My brother's girlfriend and my father programmed the head nurse to decode and talk to any important people on the phones.

> **PN:** *The professional again notes Craig's image of an all-powerful father, able to program the heads of people and having "special" ways of communicating. Note the paranoid nature of this delusion and its implications for fears of being controlled.*

My floor was being taken over by my father's close friends. My father went into one of the offices where they were having a top secret meeting about me and the girl. At the same time, I was being examined by a woman doctor. She stuck some wires on my head and kept them in place with putty. She told me to lie perfectly still while she sent my brain waves to Wisconsin for further study.

> **PN:** *Note here Craig's paranoia seems to extend into the political realm. His floor is taken over by his father's close friends. History gives us many examples of paranoid leaders purging portions of a population. For example, in the early 1950s, Joseph Stalin became convinced that there was a "doctors' plot" out to destroy him and the Soviet Union. He purged many doctors brutally, many of whom were Jews.*

While she prepared me, I asked her why she was not fastening me to the table with straps. I thought if someone were to intercept my brain waves, I would end up killing her.

> **PN:** *From a mental health vantage point, Craig becomes even more paranoid here, with aggressive impulses.*

There was a repairman outside the window now. The woman doctor calmed me down by telling me he was a guard for certain precautions. They wheeled me out in a wheelchair and positioned me next to the nurses' stations. There I acted like a deaf dumb mute person who could not understand much. While listening to the head nurse on the phone, I was able to pick up information that the enemy was closing in on the section of the hospital where I was being hidden.

The daylight was now turning into darkness. Visitors were beginning to leave. A friend of mine came with his parents to visit someone else. He was only able to see me for a few minutes.

Back in my room I was watching Archie Bunker on television. He was in a dumpy old room, playing cards at a poker table. All of a sudden I noticed Archie's voice had been changed. I began to watch the show more closely, Then I realized that they—the Mafia people with the girl—were in the room adjacent to mine. They knew they were close to me, but they were not able to get into my room because my father and I had blocked the doorway with an invisible barrier through the use of our brain waves.

Finally all hell broke out. A group of students from my high school had dressed as construction workers and were trying to free me from the hospital. They were sending me messages which the Mafia was trying to intercept. Since the Mafia had failed in accomplishing their task, they decided to have some entertainment. So the girl was programmed to kill people like a game at a penny arcade. She aimed a gun through a window and was picking off my comrades one by one.

The Nazis, at this time, began gathering all of the doctors and nurses. They lined them up outside of the hospital and starting at one end and working their way down the line, asked questions about me and the girl. They contacted my father and me and told us of their plan to execute one hostage every 10 minutes unless I was turned over to them. Now with all of this killing going on around me, I could not keep the word "kill" out of my mind. While laying in bed, if I thought the word "kill," an innocent person would be killed instantly.

> **PN:** *We should point out the further development of Craig's fantastic delusions here. He feels that the government is programmed to kill people like a game at a penny arcade. He gives himself tremendous power. If he lets the word "kill" slip out, innocent people will be killed.*
>
> *Our viewpoint is that all normal and all disturbed people have inner lives involving their own wishes, needs, conflicts, and concerns. This inner life, which everyone has, influences everyone in their daily lives but usually only influences people in a minor way. In psychosis,*

this inner life becomes elaborated, twisted up, and more extensive. In addition, it influences people to a greater amount. At times, as it mixes with the outer world, it dominates their understanding of the outer world and dominates the psychotic person (Harrow, Lanin-Kettering, Prosen, & Miller, 1983). One can see traces of this inner world and the patient's reaction and elaboration of it in the text here. Usually people monitor their behavior and thoughts, using long-term memory, with its knowledge of what the world is like, to monitor their own behavior and to help sort out the grossly unrealistic ideas (Harrow et al., 1989; Harrow & Silverstein, 1991). In psychosis, this monitoring function is ineffective. Thus, the person's use of long-term memory to help monitor and guide his/her behavior is not used effectively. This long-term memory and stored knowledge, with its ability to give an accurate estimate of the real state of the world, is still in the person's head but is not used effectively. This does not completely explain psychosis, since a number of the factors associated with psychosis are still unknown, but it does account for some of the pictures one sees here. One also can see here how the person's thoughts make sense to him/her in terms of his/her own framework, although the thoughts are still grossly unrealistic in terms of their view of the rest of the world (Frith & Corcoran, 1996; Harrow, Rattenbury, & Stoll, 1988). Thus, psychotic patients make sense in terms of their own inner framework, but one judges sanity by the realistic viewpoint of the world in general, rather than by whether an idea makes sense to the person who utters it.

While I was in the Lake City Hospital, Bob Seger's song "Still the Same" had a dramatic impact on me and still does. The following is my own breakdown of the song. ("Still the Same," written by Bob Seger, Copyright 1977 Gear Publishing Company. Permission to reprint lyrics granted by Gear Publishing, Birmingham, MI.)

You always won every time you placed a bet.

This means that it put me back to the time when all my friends and I would all gather for a friendly game of poker.

You're still damn good.

This referred to our close-knit group that made everyone feel good about one another. Even though I had this sickness, I was still their close friend and deep down, I knew I hadn't really changed.

No one's gotten to you yet.

Through all of this evil, no one has taken control over me yet.

Every time they were sure they had you caught, you were quicker than they thought.

Every time they thought they were about to catch me off guard, I was always trying to think of ways to escape their control over me.

You'd just turn your back and walk.

I would try to ignore and block out all the disturbing voices and hallucinations.

You always said, the cards would never do you wrong.

I knew there would be a way out from underneath this illness if I would just sit back in my chair and let the cards dealt to me work for me.

> **PN:** *Craig makes reference to the dramatic impact of Bob Seger's "Still the Same," a classic pop song. He interprets much of the poem in terms of trying to avoid being controlled by others and by hallucinations and voices and, finally, by illness.*

The trick you said was never play the game too long.

You've got to work this one out for yourself and don't let everything positive or negative take control of your life.

A gambler's share. The only risk you would take.

I had to take a risk on somebody to trust and believe in. This was one of the most difficult things I ever had to do. To give a part of myself to someone else and hope that the person would treat that part of me with the utmost care.

> **PN:** *Again, Craig expresses difficulties in trusting others.*

The only loss you could forsake.

The only possible thing I could do was put my trust in someone else.

The only bluff you couldn't fake. And you're still the same.

There was no hiding it. I definitely would need help from others to get through this time of confusion. "I'm still Craig deep down, trying to fight my way out." I would tell myself this to make me feel good about myself.

I caught up with you yesterday. Moving game to game. No one standing in your way.

I was beginning to take charge in trying to figure out this whole complex puzzle. And no one was going to stop me in bringing myself back into the real world.

Long enough to get you by.

I would cooperate with the hospital staff long enough to figure out what the system was and what was expected of me to get by.

You're still the same. You still aim high.

I think I aim a little too high with my goals for myself, but I still feel I have to aim high if I want to get anywhere.

There you stood. Everybody watching you play. I just turned and walked away.

It was like someone was watching over my shoulder the entire time. They were guiding me around all the barriers away from the danger and stayed long enough to see that I was just doing fine. Then just turned and walked away.

I had nothing left to say. Cause you're still the same.

I'm still Craig and no one could take that away from me.

You're still the same. Moving game to game.

I keep on moving to better myself even today.

Some things never change.

Some things never will change even though I may face horrifying experiences.

You're still the same.

I know I'm Craig and that's all that counts.

Now back to the hospital situation: A student named Mark was made up to the last detail to look and act like me. He was sent here to lure away the evil people who infested the hospital.

Meanwhile, I heard sounds in the hall as the KKK moved their massive guillotine on its wheels. It looked as if it was from around the time of Louis XVI. The KKK lined my friends up in the hall. The women were the first to go. The head man, the executioner, was seated during the long process. He would ask each victim the same questions. Each would reply—either verbally or with a motion of their head side to side—that they knew not of me. The line grew shorter as the dead bodies piled up. The executioner managed to find my brother, Alex, and a friend, Roy. The executioner assigned a couple of men to torture them to a slow, painful death. The men strapped Alex and Roy down. They selected operating tools to experiment on them. One started drilling holes into my brother's leg with a hand drill. The other began to saw Roy's left leg off. The man, if you can call him a man, that worked on my brother, sawed his right leg off. Then the two men from the Klan left Alex and Roy for dead. During the whole time, Alex and Roy wished me dead. But in the back of their minds they knew the purpose of suffering for another.

> **PN:** *Note here that a great deal of Craig's anger is manifested as delusions that the KKK was guillotining people as well as conducting bizarre medical experiments. Alex and Roy, Craig's brother and friend, were tortured for him. Each had a leg sawed off. Yet they wished him dead. The two together only had two legs. They become one person. This idea of fusing separate entities may have important psychodynamic implications.*

I was going to be taken to Cedar View Hospital. My father and mother walked me to the elevator, which would bring us to the main floor and out to the parking lot. I could hear Alex and Roy coming down the hall after us. They walked arm and arm and held themselves up; each used his own good leg to help the other walk. We left the two of them behind. The doctors were there now after the bloodshed to put people back together again. They would brainwash these victims of the incident so they could live ordinary lives again with no memory of what had happened.

My father went for his car. During his absence, a strange car pulled up and the driver offered me a ride wherever I wanted to go. I could tell this wasn't going to be easy. But I turned him down and went with my parents. I was between my folks in the front seat. The ride was like no other ride I ever had. I was able to hear some kind of sound coming from the trunk. My father was unable to keep it secret. He told me not to look back, but I knew he had saved the head of one of his top men.

> **PN:** *Note that Craig's trip to Cedar View Hospital becomes a weird adventure driving with his father who has put the head of one of his top men (who had been beheaded by a guillotine) in the trunk.*

My father drove very carefully down country roads. As he came upon an intersection, he would signal the other waiting cars with his windshield wipers. If they signaled with a reply, it was safe to further the journey.

I thought I heard something faint off in the distance. It got louder as it drew near. It was a helicopter. I grew more nervous as it flew over head. I thought it was going to open fire on us. But as strangely as it came, it left.

Finally, I arrived at Cedar View Hospital. I was told to wait in the waiting room while my father talked with some people. I felt safe and more at ease with the new people around me. I heard something going on at the entrance door of the building. The voices were from the nurses' station where a few people had gathered.

The people with whom I was sitting tried to calm me down by saying the word "relax" over and over again. It was helping until the word "kill" slipped out. A shot rang out. A person fell to the ground and so another person died because of me. The Mafia pulled their men back out of the hospital. They left the girl to plead guilty by herself, the same girl who earlier was in the Lake City Hospital and followed by the Mafia.

> **PN:** *Again from the standpoint of the mental health professional, obviously this material, as the other material, is based partly on an elaboration and twisting up of Craig's inner life. For example, Craig expresses a sense of grandiosity. He again blames himself for the deaths of innocent people by letting the word "kill" slip out. Is this a wish or a fear?*

I had been called to enter the office where my parents had been seated. The lady behind the desk asked a few questions. Then they had me sign some paper to register me into the hospital. I then was brought to another office to talk to a doctor with an odd name. As I sat comfortably in a chair, I noticed a man and a lady walking up to my parents' car and getting in. Could these be my own parents? But it couldn't be them leaving me behind. I started to lose confidence in this place.

I can't remember the name of the person who took me to my ward. I'll describe the place to you. The first thing you saw as you walked up to it was a glass wall with a door in it. The entire wall was covered with heavy metal webbing. I thought to myself, what kind of people have to be locked up in a place like that? I should have known the odds were against me when I asked that question. I entered the hall, which had rooms on both sides.

Two young men walked up to me. Neither one said a word. They just stood there with a mean glare in their eyes. I told them that they didn't look very tough to me. A nurse came to give me a pill to take. The nurse and the two young men tried to persuade me to take the pill. I refused. A few minutes went by. Then an older man came up and asked me to take down my pants so he could give me a shot. I refused again. But this time they wrestled me down on a bed to give me my shot.

I slept in a regular bed that night. I woke up the next morning, got dressed, and decided to walk around the hall to meet some people. I sat down on the floor next to this girl. She began telling me how she had seen the devil himself. Since she could see the devil, I told her I could see Jesus. We both were amazed with each others' spoken words. We talked for a while.

> **PN:** *It may be important here that Craig becomes friends with a girl. She told him she had seen the devil. He told her he had seen Jesus. Craig seems to see the world in sharp contrasts between good and evil rather then in the more subtle differentiations occurring in life.*

I got up from the floor and entered through an open door into this room. The floor had been carpeted unlike the bare, cold tile floors elsewhere. I walked around furniture to examine a record player. I began to shuffle through albums and also some old magazines. I picked up a few of the magazines and sat in a chair. I would leaf through a few pages at a time. There were messages on the pages wherever I stopped. It was just like the magazines I looked through in the Lake City Hospital waiting room. There were messages on the pages then too. While I was looking through the magazine, my eye caught hold of the massive steel door in the hall. It had a small window that had been blocked with a human heart. I read through some of the articles. I tried to figure out why some words were left out.

Gary brought me my food on a tray that he placed on the coffee table in front of the couch. Before eating, I would have to inspect the food by smelling it. After the meal, I sacked out on the couch. I was awakened by one of the nurses who told me if I wanted to sleep, I was to go to my room to do so. Now, awake, I headed for my room. Gary stopped me halfway to ask me if I would like to go for a walk on the hospital grounds. I said yes. We headed down halls unfamiliar to me. We approached the door that led to the outside world. We walked a short distance when I told him I could find my way home from here. I began to walk faster, and just as I was ready to start running, Gary grabbed me by the arm.

Gary talked me into walking back with him instead of having to force me. For not cooperating with them, I was placed in a room with a steel door and a heart in the window. The first thing I did was to tear the heart from the window. It wasn't actually a heart at all but an old dried out flower, which I flushed down the toilet.

> **PN:** *Note the richness of Craig's delusions. He first is taken for a walk. He tries to escape but is restrained by Gary (attendant) and put in a locked room with a steel door and windows. He sees a heart in the window (which turned out to be an old dried-out flower), which he tore out and flushed down the toilet.*

The room I was in had no bed; instead there was a yellow mat on the floor. There was a bathroom with a sink, a toilet, and a door. In the back of the room was a window that had been fogged on the bottom half, but it had clear glass from the middle to the top. It was all encased with metal webbing. On the ceiling was this lone light bulb surrounded by more metal webbing. There also was a fire detector.

Someone unlocked the door and entered with a food tray. He placed it on the floor next to the mat where I was sitting. I mentioned to him I didn't drink coffee and told him I wanted a coke. He left me alone while I finished my meal. I started to get mad about being locked in this place. I stood with my back to the metal door. Then I began to pound on the door and yell at the top of my lungs. My hands began to hurt with this pulsating pain. I stopped for a second, then I sang anything that came into my mind, mostly church songs that I made up at the time. The young man, who brought me my dinner, opened the door and presented me with a coke. He positioned himself on the floor across from me. In his hand was a second can, a coke. He talked with me while we drank. As I was almost done with my drink, I shook the can with a few drops at the bottom. Then, I had no way of knowing how he did it, but I had a half can of coke to drink again. He struck me as a person whom I could trust. I asked him if he could find me a pillow and a blanket for the night. He presented me with them both and said that, if I cooperated, they would find me another room.

I was awakened the next morning by a noise that sounded like helicopters landing and taking off. By pulling myself up with my fingers around the metal caging, I tried to see through the clear part of the window. Then I tried a different approach by grabbing the top of the bathroom door and pulling myself up far enough to get my feet on the door knobs. By looking out the window, I spotted a riding lawn mower which was making the sounds of my imaginary helicopters.

> **PN:** *Note Craig's continued resistance and delusions.*

"Time for breakfast," Gary said as he pulled his key out of the lock. He had me follow him out from the caged-in hallway. We walked on by the nurses' station to this kitchen, which could have fit in anyone's home. Gary had me select a few items from the refrigerator, but I could only take the ones without name tags on them. I walked over to a table and sat down to eat my fruit and drink my milk. I noticed a nurse, whose voice really traveled, talking. She was talking to these patients about going for a ride in the country. I thought that would be a good way to get out of this place for a while. So I walked over to the desk and signed my name to the list.

Gary found me out in the hall and asked if I was finished eating. I answered yes, so he asked me if I'd like to watch some television. I answered yes again. There were quite a few old people in the sitting room. I thought I recognized one lady as my grandmother, but I didn't talk to her because I thought she was put here to watch over me and protect me.

I went out in the hall, without Gary seeing me, then down the hall until I came upon a pay telephone. I seated myself on this wooden stool and began to dial a series of numbers. The operator kept cutting in on me. Finally, I got the right sequence of numbers, and I heard ringing now. Someone answered. It was my mother. It was pleasing to hear a familiar voice again. I only had a few short moments to talk to her, but it was refreshing.

> **PN:** *Again it is important to note the power of Craig's mother's voice.*

On my way back to the ward, Gary came upon me and walked me back to the caged-in area. I had privileges. For example, I could wander back and forth between my room and the room I had visited the day before. I entered that well-furnished room. I picked up a deck of playing cards off a table, sank down in an easy chair, shuffled the cards, and placed them in order on the foot stool for a game of solitaire. I didn't play by the normal rules; instead of playing every third card, I played every card. After the game, I fell asleep on the couch.

I was awakened by a nurse who presented me with a tray of food for dinner. She told me if I wanted to sleep, I was to do it in my own room. When I had finished eating, I decided to see if I was able to find someone to talk to. I found a room with the door open, so I walked in. There propped up with pillows on a bed was this small man reading a book. I asked him if he would mind if I talked to him. He said that he wouldn't mind. We talked for a few minutes. Then he picked up his book, readjusted his pillow, and started to read again. As I left, I said, "See you later" and walked over to a room with special furniture. I found out later that room was a meeting room for doctors, nurses, and staff.

Back in my room, I stretched out on my mat. There was silence throughout the room. As I lay there motionless, I heard foot steps in the hall, followed by a knock at my door. The door was unlocked and swung open. There stood a nurse with pills I had to take. As the nurse left, I hadn't noticed that Gary was there also. Gary asked me if I would like to shower and shave. I answered with a yes. I picked out some clean clothes from a closet just outside the caged-in hall.

Gary led me into a room where two men in single beds were sleeping. He said they wouldn't mind me using the bathroom. Gary told me to shave and then shower down while he looked for some dry towels. I shaved, but I hesitated about taking a shower. Gary returned with towels and asked why I hadn't showered yet. I thought to myself—if I get into the shower stall, I might get severely burned. Gary tested the water and told me to hurry up with my shower. I took the shower and changed into clean clothes.

Late that night, a man rushed into my room. He woke me up and hurried me through a smoke-filled hall. I went past the nurses' station. Then the man told me to sit down in the television room. I was a little shaken up by all of this. As I was watching television, I noticed a piece of driftwood on one of the shelves. At the time, it looked as if it were an arm that had been burned to a crisp. The man who took me out of my room eventually brought me back to it. He told me there might be a little smell of smoke but it would be safe for me to sleep now.

> **PN:** *Note that Craig is still delusional. He sees driftwood as an arm that was burnt to a crisp.*

Morning came fast because of the interruption during the night. The guy who brought me a coke entered my room with my breakfast. It was the end of his shift, but he wanted to tell me I was going to be transferred to another building sometime today. This was surprising considering what I had done. I was mad at them for putting me in a place like this, so I decided to try to flood my room. I noticed the pipes below the sink. I placed my feet on the wall and pulled with all of my strength on one of the pipes. The pipe moved, then water leaked out in a slow steady stream. When the nurse came in to give me my pills, she noticed the puddle forming on the floor. I took the pills. Then she told me to go into the room where they had their meetings while she got someone to fix the leak.

> **PN:** *Note the potentially destructive aspects of the patient's thought disorder. He tried to flood the room by breaking the sink.*

Soon I was going to another building. I was thinking of this while lying on my mat staring at the ceiling, when I heard someone rapping on my door. I rose to my feet and walked over to the door. I looked through my window and all I could see were two eyes staring back at me. He said he loved me, and I replied I love you too if you can get me out.

I was still in the same building a bit longer. Breakfast went fast because I think I was getting used to the type of food they serve here. I kept telling them that I don't drink coffee, but I set it aside for my father in case he would stop by. He drank the coffee that I used to set aside in the Lake City Hospital. I walked over to the easy chair and picked up the cards and started preparing them for a mean game of solitaire. About half way through the deck, the cards were in my favor, and then out of the corner of my eye I caught a glimpse of a girl who looked about my age or younger. She walked in; we exchanged names. Marge was her name. Marge then sat down and started fidgeting with her purse. She was talking to her purse as if it could hear her voice. I just sat there with my card game even though she thought her purse was more interesting than me.

A nurse stopped in to see if Marge would like to go for a walk on the hospital grounds. The nurse said I had some visitors waiting to see me. In walked my mother and father. I asked how the cats, the dog, and Alex were doing. My mother had a bag with coin magazines and a large bag of peanuts inside, but they could only stay for a short while.

After visiting with my parents, I took a nap. I was awakened by one of the nurse's aides. He said they had someone I'd probably like to talk to. I'll call him Bob. I thought that he was one of the President's secret service men. I thought he had come to talk with me before I would meet with the President to tell him my story. Bob seemed to know quite a bit about my home town. I had to stop thinking about things that weren't true. I had to start listening to people before I began to judge them. Bob, it turns out, was from Lake City and was in the hospital for his own reasons. We talked about Lake City High School and the different teachers we had.

Gary told me he would help me gather my things because I'd be moving into another building this afternoon. I don't remember how I left the Warren build-ing or how I got into the Augustus building. I remember sitting down on my suitcase and bending it out of shape in the hallway of the Augustus building.

Then, this strange, tall fellow came up to me and started tapping me in the chest with his fingers while he asked me what my name was. I replied, "Craig," and then I asked him his name while I began tapping him on the chest. He said, "I'm Milo," while he stood teetering back and forth. I couldn't understand how he was able to sway that way without falling over.

A nurse found me in the hall, with my suitcase. She had me follow her to a room where I was to bed down with two older men. There was also one empty bed for a future patient.

The Augustus building is the oldest building on the grounds. Cedar View Hospital has many types of buildings and areas. There is the Warren Therapy Center, an Adolescent Center, offices, a chapel, half-way houses, workshops, baseball diamonds, and a man-made pond with a variety of birds around it.

The first few days I spent sitting on a footstool in the front foyer of the Augustus building. I would sit and try to figure things out. People would come in and out all day long. I would sit there on my stool between the coats that were dangling all around me from the coat rack above. I would watch very closely to learn the system of entering and leaving the building. To enter, you have to knock, ring the bell, or use your key if you had your own pass key. To leave, you had to find a person with a key in order to exit. The people would smile and greet me with a "hello." I replied the same way. I tried several times to slip out the door while people entered or left the building. But my attempts were not successful.

The days spent at the Augustus building started out with a wake-up call, which meant that it was time for breakfast soon so you had to be and dressed and ready to eat. Breakfast was served in a small dining room where the trays were brought from one of the larger buildings that had a bigger and more equipped kitchen.

Each day would be planned out ahead of time in the Augustus building. They had different events going on all day long. There were Bible classes, goals group, cooking class, relaxation group, and discussion group. Outdoor activities were also held outside the Augustus building for recreation or free time.

I went to Bible class only a few times. It was the same for me with chapel on Sundays and sing-alongs. Goals group was basically spent thinking up goals for yourself for your week ahead. If you couldn't think of a goal, the group would help you out with suggestions for a goal. You also had to tell the group if you thought you had accomplished your goal from the week before.

As patients, we were all required to plan out certain time slots in the day and fill them in with how we would like to spend that time. Our weekends were planned by the staff. Cooking class required that we plan a menu for either breakfast, lunch, or dinner once a week. We purchase all the ingredients from the grocery store across the street. On the second floor of the Augustus building there was a small kitchen where we all chipped in preparing and cooking the meal.

Our relaxation group would all gather in one room where we listened to a tape with suggested relaxation techniques. Our group would all lie on our backs and totally relax our bodies, by relaxing one part of our body at a time. Some of us are in the relaxation state while others have fallen asleep.

Exercise was a class that didn't last because of lack of interest. In discussion groups, you deal with your feelings in many different ways. Everyone tells about whatever comes to mind. They tell their feelings about different situations and how they came to be in the Augustus building. They reveal their present feelings about themselves and how they feel about the people around them. We tell how we think we will feel when we are out of the hospital. Also, we make comments on one another to see them progressing or regressing.

Our recreation and free time consisted in the use of the gym in the Warren building where we played basketball, volleyball, and other games. In the summer, we played outdoors on the baseball diamonds. To be trusted to leave the building on our own was a special privilege we had to earn. After proving that we were responsible, we were allowed the use of bicycles on our own, and we also were able to go to and from the store.

The best part of all was being allowed to leave the Augustus building and walk over to the Warren building for lunch or dinner. It was nice to be able to eat with different people, which would give me a break from the people I would see day in and day out. The neat thing is that everyone ate in the same dining room: patients, doctors, nurses, therapists, and secretaries. The food really tasted good. We also would go there for our ice cream outings or some-times to Tom's Ice Cream Snack Shop down the road on Division Avenue.

We went on many outings away from the facility, such as picnics, roller skating, garage sales, shopping in the malls, and various other activities.

> **PN:** *Note that Craig has begun to adjust to his environment. He be-gins to join groups. He goes to Bible classes. He seemingly becomes well enough to leave the facility. He goes out on car rides but now tries to escape from the van in traffic. He even begins to make some friends. His perceptions of these people, while sketchy, are not without insight.*

Now I'm going to tell you some stories about the people I got to know.

Jack, a black worker, was a pretty nice guy once you got to know him. One day while we were out for a van ride, there was an accident up ahead on Twenty-eighth Street. The van started to move up to the traffic signal. I jumped out of the van while it started to move with the traffic. The driver stopped the van and Jack jumped out after me. He caught up with me and asked me where I was headed. I said I wanted to see if I could help. Jack walked me back to the van. From that point on, everyone had to wear safety belts and the doors had to be locked.

Betsy is a blonde worker. It's hard to say if blondes have more fun, especial-ly at the Augustus building. One day I got back a little late from a meet-ing I had with a man named Ben. Betsy had already started her crafts class. I entered and quietly took my place at a wooden bench where I was to make designs in leather work. Betsy was over at the sink helping someone with a problem. I had to use a hammer to stamp out designs in leather. I decided to let her know I was there, so I swung the hammer around and brought it forcefully down on the table, making a sound that echoed throughout the room. You should have seen the way Betsy jumped into the air. When she landed, this little lady had come alive with anger, which was focused on me. She started rattling off. . . .

I also met people in the television room. Sitting and watching television was a major pastime. The chairs, in a variety of colors, were set in an L shape in front of the television. Something is always happening around the television. A lady named Wilhelmina would sit and feed the dog, Pepper, cigarette butts from her ashtray, a practice the nurses frowned upon. Wilhelmina would start screaming if she didn't get an extra cigarette, beyond the limit of cigarettes allowed each day from the nurses' station.

Chester, one of the workers, would tease Wilhelmina by holding a cigarette a few inches from her mouth. Then she would try to grab it with her lips. It was a funny sight to see. It was amazing how Chester could move around the building. One minute he was sitting next to you watching television; the next minute he was gone. Then you would look around again and see him sitting a couple of chairs away, watching television again. Chester was like a magician the way he could move so quietly and fast, popping up here and there— sometimes without your even knowing it.

Chester has long hair that reaches down his back and a mustache over his upper lip. He dresses in blue jeans and a tee shirt, with a pocket that held his Camel short cigarettes. Visitors and patients alike couldn't tell that he was part of the staff.

Hank is an old man from the other wing of the building where the older people live—like in many old people's homes. He has a voice that can echo and travel with ear piercing noise throughout the halls. You have to be careful of what you might do or say around Hank because you are never quite sure how he might react. Chester, however, was always under control when dealing with Hank. Chester seems to have a way with all people in the Augustus building. He has a subtle humor that has always tickled my funny bone. This entertainment was just what everyone needed to cheer up.

One day Hank was watching television and had to leave his chair to go to the restroom. When he returned, he noticed that his seat had a small puddle of water on it. He then went and returned and dried his chair with paper towels. He threw the towels away, returned again, sat down, then bounced back up and proceeded to dry his chair once again. This went on a couple of times until he caught Chester at wetting his chair. With his wrinkled brow and squashed, upturned nose, Hank raced around the pool table chasing Chester and limping at the same time. Chester, mocking Hank's limp, stayed in front, just out of reach. Hank tired and so did his anger weaken towards Chester.

Shooting pool was one of my favorite pastimes. I usually took Chet on in a game of pool when he had time. It was a challenge playing Chester because he used sleight of hand. You always had to keep an eye on him because if you took your eye off the table for one minute, usually more of your pool balls and less of his were on the playing table. You had to keep track of both: how many balls you and he had on the table. You also had to keep track of him because he was somewhere behind you, usually moving the balls in and out of the pockets or into impossible positions for your next shot.

Medication was given a few times a day; everyone had to line up in front of the nurses' station. My pills consisted of a few blue pills and a couple of white pills. The blue ones are stelazine, and the white ones are cogentin. Stelazine slows you way down, makes you tired, blurs your vision, and dries out your mouth. Cogentin is used to counteract the muscle spasms that you can get from the stelazine. The stelazine is a major tranquilizer for schizophrenia. I found myself more tired than usual. My vision was most difficult in reading or doing fine, detailed work.

My doctor is a lady, Dr. Stanley, who had an office in the Warren building. She gave me a few little tests. One had to do with counting. Another had to do with the meaning of phrases. One phrase was "People in glass houses shouldn't throw stones," for which I was to come up with an explanation or answer to see if it's normal. Then the doctor would hold my arm at my forearm and bend my arm in an upward motion at my elbow. My doctor would meet with me every so often through my stay at Cedar View, basically to change my medication when needed. I also had a psychologist named Ted Thatcher who met with me quite a bit. When I met with Ted, I usually didn't talk much to him. He would sit with his legs propped up on his desk while biting on his tongue. We both would sit there staring at each other. He'd ask me a few questions, and then I'd ask him a few questions. We'd both run out of things to say, and we would agree to end our session early for a trip to the dining room for some ice cream.

The other patients around me had problems of their own, but I really don't remember what they were. Ray Jasper was a different sort of person. He always carried a notebook with all kinds of drawings on space flights and satellites in it. It also contained information on military jets. He looked so important carrying this thick notebook around with him wherever he went. Once in a while, I'd go up to his room and we'd listened to his *Beatles* record album collection.

Milo was the strangest of all the residents. One time he started pestering me because I hadn't eaten all of my dinner. He looked over the top of his glasses while shaking his finger at me and said "Geiser, Geiser, eat the rest of your food, Geiser." Then I would reply in his tone of voice, "Milo, Milo, mind your own business, Milo."

Once we all gathered to play a game of softball at one of the diamonds. Milo was on the opposite team. I was the pitcher when Milo approached the plate for his time up at bat. Milo wasn't one of the better ball players on his team, but he tried awful hard to hit that ball. I carefully watched where Milo was swinging his bat when I pitched him the ball over the plate. He still missed the first two pitches. I fed him the third ball which just happened to connect with his bat. You should have been there to see everyone's reaction to him hitting the ball! The ball he hit dribbled a couple of feet from the pitcher's mound. His team members were all cheering and yelling for him to run to first base. Milo made it safe to first base, with a little help from me. My team members were in an uproar at me for not throwing him out. I think anyone in my position would have done the same for Milo.

Whenever we went out of the building and Milo was coming along with us, everyone would say, "Let's go Milo." One time while going to an event, Milo was riding in the back of the bus and I was following with another group in a car. Milo would sit facing forward with his head turned sideways watching us with one eye during the whole trip.

We were all at a music event in a park one evening, sitting on a picnic table. Milo was over to one side of the table tapping his foot and snapping his fingers to the music. Everyone got more enjoyment from watching him than from the musicians who were there to entertain us.

Jenny was a worker in the housekeeping department. She was one of my favorites, and she was very kind to me. She would do little extra things to make my stay as comfortable as possible. She showed me how to open and close the windows to cool or warm up the room. She would bring me a fan when it was hot and blankets when the weather got cold. She found me a small closet to store my clothes in so I wouldn't have to live out of my suitcase anymore. There was a time that I wouldn't unpack my suitcase because I didn't want to think I was going to stay any length of time.

There was this older gentleman named Hector who wore a distinguished long, graying beard on his aging face. Hector took me for a mystical man with certain powers that were not understood by the ordinary. He would intrigue me as he would stare straight out into space and make these hand motions as though he were picking something evil right out of the air before him and discarding it back across the room from where it had come. He would grow with anger as this evil presence began bombarding him from all directions. Hector then would look up to the ceiling and reach out with one arm stretched out as if grasping something from above. And then he would bring his arm down in a slow, jagged motion as If pulling a barrier down around himself. The evil then would vanish from his presence, and he would fall fast asleep in an armchair in front of the television.

Cedar View was confusing me the way they could change the looks of a building in one day. They could paint an entire building or put in a new sidewalk in one day, it seemed to me. Something always was being changed. On the insides of buildings, they were adding rooms or moving rooms around. The way I was thinking made it hard to understand these changes.

> **PN:** *One can note that the changes at Cedar View are very confusing to Craig—whether it is the painting a building or putting in a sidewalk.*

I wanted to be released from Cedar View. You have to prove that you are ready. Your medication plays a big part in this. At first you are able to go home on weekends to see how well you do in the community and to see if you take your medicine on schedule. The first thing I wanted to do when I was released was for my brother to drive me around in my Opal GT. The doctor wanted me to come back for visits and checkups at Cedar View. After a few times back there, I talked her into letting me see her in Lake City for medication changes. I've also been seeing a psychologist on a regular basis. I was released from Cedar View near the end of the month of August, 1978.

There are many adverse reactions to my medicine. This is what the *Physicians' Desk Reference, Fortieth Edition* (1986) says: Cogentin (white tablet small) Adverse Reactions: Dry mouth, blurred vision, nausea and nervousness may develop. If dry mouth is severe, there is difficulty in swallowing or speaking, or loss of appetite and weight. Vomiting occurs infrequently. Occasionally, an allergic reaction, skin rash develops. Stelazine (blue tablet) Adverse Reactions: Drowsiness, dizziness, skin reaction, rash, dry mouth, Insomnia, amenorrhea, fatigue, muscular weakness, anorexia, lactation, blurred vision and neuromuscular reactions (extrapyramidal).

> **PN:** *One might note that Craig read the Physician's Desk Reference possibly to get a list of adverse reactions to medication. Perhaps this is Craig's way of obtaining some sort of control.*

When I was released, most of my time was spent readjusting myself to the people around me, especially to my parents and my brothers. Actually I spent most of the time sleeping. From what I understand, basically, the medication made me drowsy. I've been meeting with psychiatrists, psychologists, and social workers, including Dr. Stanley, through this whole period, and today I'm still seeing them. I would meet with Dr. Stanley every three months for a checkup and also to renew my prescription. I also met with a psychologist whose name is Fred Garr.

I was nervous when I entered the Community Mental Health Clinic in Lake City for my first time. Fred Garr was a straightlaced, every-hair-in-place type of guy. In the back of my mind, I was wondering if Fred was going to be a carbon copy of Ted Thatcher. It took a little while for Fred and I to break the ice and for me to ease back in my chair. The conversation began to flow, and it wasn't as one-sided as I had encountered with Ted. Fred would throw in bits of information—which would help me out of my stalemate—to keep the ball rolling. The thing I liked most about Fred was that he let me ask any questions I might have, like how things were going today or even personal things dealing with his life.

After my meeting with the psychologist, I would visit with Dr. Stanley. I was always trying to persuade her to lower my prescription dosage, and I was always pressing and prying to find out when I would no longer have to take my medicine. Every so often she would lower my dosage. This made me feel as if I was on my way to being cured. No one ever told me that I was schizophrenic or really sat down and explained to me what was going on inside of me. It wasn't until I was hospitalized in Cedar View for a second time that it was explained to me in a brief way that I was classed as a schizophrenic.

Soon I was being tested to see where my interests lay for a career. My highest interest was in art, followed by floor covering. For practical reasons, I was encouraged to seek a career in floor covering. I guess they thought I wouldn't be able to make a living as an artist. I was to take more testing to see if I qualified for the floor covering program at the State Rehabilitation Center.

The State Rehabilitation Center had the atmosphere of a college setting. It was out in the countryside, next to a small lake that was connected to a few other lakes by channels. The grounds were pretty—with wild flowers and trees. There were basketball courts, tennis courts, and a baseball diamond. Inside the building there were three floors of dorm rooms, one side for men and the other side for women. They had classrooms at one end and a huge cafeteria at the other end of the building.

There were many things one could do for recreation in the building. One was playing pool. Pool is one of my favorite types of recreation. It was quite different shooting pool with the people staying there. I've shot pool with a man there in a wheelchair. That isn't easy. Another time I played pool with a short guy who used two crutches with which he used to propel himself all over the facility on a skateboard. He would hop up on the pool table and shoot a game.

The facility had an Olympic-size pool. I saw the national champion of the wheelchair swimmers swimming in the pool.

There was a paraplegic woman who swam the width of the pool by her breathing according to this one man. If I hadn't seen some of these things, they would have been hard to believe.

One time I was in the archery range and watched a man getting ready to shoot at a target. As he pulled back and shot, I noticed that he was different. He was crippled in one arm. He would somehow pull back the string with the arrow by using his teeth and then firing it, but he hit the target anyway.

The facility's bowling alleys were equipped with bowling ball ramps that enabled the wheelchair people to maneuver the ball.

In addition, there was a room used for leather crafts and one for ceramics. There were all kinds of places to spend your time after classes. The facility came equipped with a huge gymnasium and a library.

The Rehabilitation Center tested for many types of career choices. We could choose a few. My choices were clock and watch repair, jewelry, drafting, and floor covering. The outcome of my testing showed that I had a high score in floor covering. I was to start State Rehabilitation after the holidays in January, 1979.

When I attended classes at State Rehabilitation, I met this guy named Peter. We started getting together after class and became close friends. Peter was humorous. He would find humor in ordinary things in an original way that would put a smile on everyone. We need each other emotionally just as we need vitamins for our well-being. Peter provided some of this emotional support for me. I kept in touch with Peter. When I began at State Rehabilitation, I was given a roommate, Rex. I had become friends with everyone in class, especially Cliff.

> **PN:** *Craig seemed to be improving. He began to participate in the floor covering program at the State Rehabilitation Center. He began to appreciate that other people experience difficulties.*

One day the whole process started happening again with my thoughts. It seemed as though everyone I had passed in the hall on to class was calling my name out. I would hear, "Craig," and I would turn to see who it was and then someone else would call out my name until everybody I passed was saying my name under their breaths. I figured out for myself that this rehabilitation center was here because of me. All these people were being rehabilitated back into society with new careers from my stay in Lake City Hospital where all the killings and mishaps had taken place.

> **PN:** *We must emphasize here Craig's second psychotic break. He started becoming paranoid again. He felt everyone was calling his name out again. Craig drew picture of man from the Middle East with a Roman nose. It looked as if he were from a religious cult. One can see again how part of Craig's inner life, and elaborations of it, begin to dominate his thinking.*

While waiting out in the hall for my class to begin, a lady walked by with a briefcase and informed me everything was okay and I was safe. I knew I was to be leaving The State Rehab soon. That day in class they needed my booth for a student to take his linoleum cutting test. I was to read up on my next project while waiting for an open booth. While seated at the table, I began staring at my hand intensely. I laid my hand on the table, palm down. With my concentration focused on my hand, it was as if I could move my hand and fingers with thoughts from my brain. I picked up my pen and drew a picture. It was as if another force was guiding my pen across the paper. The picture I drew was of a man from the Middle East with a Roman nose. The hat on his head looked as if it was from a religious cult. He was dressed with a long tunic and had bare feet. He had one arm stretched out with his fingers spread, and his other arm was bent at the elbow with his hand formed to a peace symbol from the sixties. I thought that this man was telling me that the peace in the world was not very stable. Also, I thought he was telling me people were beginning to build up forces to rebel against me.

One of the students put a big gash in his thumb with a utility knife. I walked over to the booth where he had been working. The utility knife lay there with blood stains on the blade. As I was looking at the knife, it turned to silver before my eyes. I asked to be excused from class to see the school nurse and doctor.

> **PN:** *Craig again becomes delusional here.*

The doctor did not believe in my paranoid thoughts. I would not trust anyone. The doctor brought in my counselor. My counselor was able to comfort me by telling me she believed what I had been telling them was not a joke or a made-up story. She told me it was noon and I could join the rest for lunch in the dining room.

While I was eating lunch, I began looking around and I noticed all of the deaf people watching me. Then I heard some voices that were trying to put me at ease with words of comfort and understanding. I looked up from another bite to realize they all had been talking to me through thought and not by words passed from mouth to ear.

After lunch I headed for my room and began packing everything in my room because I knew my father would want me to do so. I also knew that I had to pack every last thing of mine in order that no one knew that I had ever been there at the State Rehabilitation. My mother and father came to get me. I thought that they were going to take me home, but they were bringing me back to Cedar View.

> **PN:** *Note that Craig is hospitalized again at Cedar View. Now Craig has a gap in his narrative of seven years (or since his last hospitalization). During his second hospitalization he begins to think of himself as schizophrenic.*

Following my time at Cedar View, I got a job at a fast-food restaurant. I also met a woman who I thought I would be spending the rest of my life with. We went on an Autumn honeymoon to a beautiful resort in northern Michigan located on Lake Michigan. Soon we had a little boy who is the joy of my life.

> **PN:** *A gap of seven years occurs here. Then Craig continues with his narration.*

It has been seven years since the last time I had been hospitalized. I have found that it takes a while to climb back up to the mainstream. I consider myself very lucky to have such good friends, a comforting family, and such encouraging fellow workers, all who have helped me on my journey from one stepping stone to the next. I feel it has been a very positive learning experience for me. It has helped me in opening up myself to being stronger and enabled me to handle the very difficult experiences and situations society has to dish out.

> **PN:** *After seven years, one can note that Craig indicates he is better. Craig praises his comforting family. He feels his experiences opened him up to being stronger.*

I have finally found the key that had been most helpful to me in figuring out this mystery that I had been walking through. After a month of phoning, I have been able to obtain my personal files from both hospitals I stayed in. After reading them, I now have both points of view on my experience, my own and the professional view of the hospitals.

When someone asked me to explain schizophrenia, I tell them I have a way of making them understand it. I tell them: You know how sometimes you are in your dreams yourself, and some of them feel like real nightmares? Most people can relate to this. Then I tell them: It was like I was walking through a dream but everything around me was real. At times, today's world seems so boring and I wonder if I would like to step back into the schizophrenic dream, but then I remember all the scary and horrifying experiences.

> **PN:** *It is important to note that Craig tries to explain schizophrenia. "You know how sometimes you are in your dreams yourself, and some of them can feel like real nightmares? It was like I was walking through a dream but everything around me was real."*

My school yearbook reminds me of the comforts of reality. This is one of the letters in it from one of my friends: Flag (my nickname), "Boy, we sure have had a lot of good times. Like skiing, golfing, going to the beach, and just cruising or bumming around. Remember when we got stuck out by the water plant? Looking back on it, we had a good time trying to get out. We also had a lot of fun in your boat skiing and just riding around. It was good seeing you at the fair. I lost a lot of money there, trying to win a stuffed animal and I didn't even get one. Craig, you are a good friend and I'll see you again soon."

I had been married for seven years when my wife wanted a divorce. I have a little boy that I see on weekends. I enjoy having him around. He picks up my spirits. We've done all kinds of fun things together. Going camping is one of our favorites. I love filming him. He's growing up so fast!

I have been living with my parents since the divorce. It's OK, but I can't wait until I have a place of my own. I'd love to have a farm house with about 40 acres. I probably only will be able to afford a mobile home. I miss having a yard to mow and landscape.

I hope to get married again someday to a woman who can share her time, companionship, and love. This lady will like walks along Lake Michigan beaches as the sun sets in the west. She would have to understand that I'm a shy and quiet man who get nervous around beautiful women. One of the most important requirements is to have the commitment to one another for the rest of our lives.

My artwork is where I release a lot of emotions and ideas. It's relaxing for me to draw. During my 1994 hospital stay, I started incorporating color into my pictures. I get satisfied by showing my pictures to people and getting their feedback.

My feelings about myself now are hard to think about because I have such high hopes. I'm not sure if I'll reach my expectations for myself. In all, its been a big adjustment with both the divorce and the schizophrenia. I think that as the days go by I'm getting better. My medication has helped bring me back to reality with only one visible side effect: shakiness. I've come to deal with that.

I believe God has entered my life more and more. I may not go to regular church services, but I attend a church group called Dynamics In Living. In this group, we share what has been happening in our lives. We have guest speakers whose topics relate to the mentally ill. We have prayer at the beginning and finish with group prayer for anyone among us who might need help. I don't feel comfortable around large groups. And I find my needs are met through this small group.

> **PN:** *In the pages that follow, Craig has presented, from his own view-point, the very painful experience of his breakup with his wife and some further psychosis.*

Back in the fall of 1993. I experienced a good and safe bright light after I prayed to Jesus with the promise of my soul to God. It was like the morning Son shining through my bedroom window. My little boy and I were the only ones home that night. I usually say the Our Father to myself before I sleep. I asked God to bless my wife, my little boy, and myself. I especially asked God to watch over us as we slept that night. I felt as if I was saved like the Christians say. But a few days later while taking a bath, I noticed a burning sensation on my lower legs, identical patches on both legs as if I had a sunburn with no hair in those areas (unexplainable).

> **PN:** *One can note the intermingling of religious and psychotic themes. Craig experiences delusions of "lachryma Christi" (the blood of Christ), a traditional Christian belief associated mostly with Catholic Europe then with America. Burning sensations on his legs are like the wounds of Christ. He goes from being beneficiary of Christ's death (being "saved*

like the Christians say") to being Christ the martyr himself. Craig shows some thought slippage here. He misspells "sun" as "son" (Son is Jesus)— "the morning Son shining through my bedroom window."

Later in the mail, I received a chain letter that explained to me that if I mail out to 10 friends identical letters it could bring me good luck (like winning the lotto). But if I didn't follow the instructions in the letter, I could lose my job or even die. I thought I could use some good luck in my life. But then I began to think that we couldn't really afford to mail out all those letters and why should I put guilt on my friends to do the same with this chain letter within 72 hours?

A few days later I received a call on the telephone from my boss instructing me that I had to switch my work hours. They would not coincide with my wife's job. I was caught in a catch-22. Within five minutes on the phone, my six years of work with this company was over. I then proceeded to apply for unemployment. I followed all the procedures to collect. My boss told me to find another job or consider myself as being laid off. For weeks no money came in. I decided to try the temporary service and received a factory job on the second shift. I worked a good two months at the factory and still was not hired in.

PN: *Craig loses his job to accommodate his wife's work schedule, then she tells him she wants to leave. Obviously this increases his overall distress.*

About the last weekend in January, my wife and I got into an argument with one another. The anger within me came out because of my wife's vulgar language which she used with me on the phone. She said "I'm not going to get into another fucking argument on the phone." I didn't want to argue with her, but when she got home it developed into an argument. I told my little boy Matthew what the vulgar word "fuck" meant. Because she's always telling me she can talk any way she damn well pleases.

It hurts a lot inside me to write this down on paper or to talk about this because I love my wife and son very very much. I'm crying while I write this to whomever may read this in order to help me in my need to release my emotions. For better or for worse, that is the question I ask myself over and over, again and again. Divorce: Law, a judicial declaration dissolving a marriage in whole or in part. Judicial Separation: any formal separation of man and wife according to established custom. Total separation, disunion: a divorce between thought and action to break the marriage contract between oneself and one's spouse by divorce. To separate or isolate to obtain a legal divorce. My wife used this word while telling me she didn't love me anymore. Please tell me she didn't say it. Anything in the world but that word Divorce? Did she really say it? It can't be? Not me of all people? I love her. Does she know what she's saying to me? I don't know how to respond. Where did that come from? She's said it before? Does she really mean what she's saying to me? I feel like the rug is been pulled out from under my feet. Everything is racing through my mind right now. I begin to shake and tremble inside. I withdraw into my chair. Every thing becomes foggy through my tearful sight of my wife and son. I can't stop crying. I cover my eyes. I wish I could disappear. What to do? What to do? I'm scared. What's going to happen to me? My little boy Matthew? What about him? She's been thinking about this for a while. I haven't. Do I leave or does she? I've got to leave; it hurts too much to stay. I need some money and clothes. She suggests I stay at my folks house since they are on vacation down south. She has nowhere to go, so it's up to me to leave. She lets me take the car since she could walk to work. Her friend is going to take care of Matthew when she's working. We were helping her friend out by letting her stay with us because she's going to get a divorce from her husband. Deja vu or what? I used the phone to call someone who might be home to talk to. My uncle was home and said I could come over to talk.

I filled the car up with gas and left Forest View around 5 p.m. in a light winter snow. The drive seemed to take forever. "St. Peter thank God I'm here." Getting out of the car was kind of hard. I felt weak-kneed and wobbly. My uncle greeted me at the door. I told him I felt like I was on jet lag and that when I walked it felt as though I was two feet above the ground. I felt so light and disoriented. I asked for a beer and sat down behind a plant which was on the table. My uncle missed his dinner appointment but was kind enough to stay with me and talk. Hiding behind the plant, I felt ashamed with the predicament I got myself into. After talking for a while and relieving some of my hurt, I was able to come out from hiding.

I joined him for dinner in town. After talking a while I was beginning to feel better, right? I felt I was being torn apart in all different directions with the questions again. What to do? What to do? Brenda, Matthew, Uncle Don, family, in-laws, and the hardest one of all, myself?

I departed that late evening by myself to make it home though the lonely cold winter night. What is fair? What is right? How will this look for others who perceive us as a perfect couple? Who cares what others think? I love Brenda and Matthew. "I don't know anymore how to prove to Brenda and Matthew how much I really do love them both, more than anything in the world.

I've been racking my brain over and over and over. I'm to the point of self-destruction or brain overload, Dust in the wind, Dust in the wind." I keep moving on. In what direction? I'm not sure yet?

I arrive home. No one there. Good, maybe I can put this behind me, that this never happened, like a bad dream. Wrong, I'm still hiding and hurting within. Where's Brenda and Matthew? That's right, Matthew's at the in-laws tonight and Brenda was going to party with friends tonight. 11:00 pm went to bed. Bam! Bam! Bam! Knock, knock, knock, "I'm coming, I'm coming." I look through the blinds; it's Sandy. The door flings open she looks drunk I don't say anything and go back to bed. She uses the bathroom then heads back outside. Midnight. Car door shuts, loud, car backs out of driveway and sits in the street. I had gotten up to look. Thought maybe Sandy and Brenda were mad at me and were going to try to sleep in the car all night. I go back to bed.

> **PN:** *One can note that Craig engages in denial. He hopes he can make this (the divorce) never happen like a bad dream. Craig is worried that his wife and her girlfriend are mad at him.*

1 o'clock ring, ring, ring. Half asleep, I answer the phone. There is laughing on the other end of the phone. I thought this must be Sandy because of the drunken giggling. It was the gal who threw the party. She wanted to know if Brenda and Sandy made it home all right. I told her about the car outside and that I'd check it out and tell them to come in the house to sleep after saying thanks. I open the blinds. No car. Now what do I do? I tried to find that girl's number in the address book? No luck. So I called my in-laws because I was worried Brenda and Sandy might be drunk riding around at night in the snow. Brenda's mother answered, and I explained to her what was going on. She said she had the phone number and would take care of it and not to worry and try to get some sleep. I said I was sorry to wake her but I didn't know what to do.

I received a phone call from Brenda this morning. I answered. She told me a different story about what had happened last night with my phone calling around, and I proceeded to tell her she must not have been listening to the people she had gotten her information from. Not easy talking to Brenda on the phone. I then proceeded to tell her that if we wanted to make this marriage work out then we would have to work at it as a family and that Sandy was going to have to move out. She then proceeded to tell me that we both agreed to have her move in on a temporary basis. I agreed, but things have changed and I didn't want her living with us anymore. I said we both agreed but I had changed my mind. Brenda didn't agree with me and proceeded to tell me my opinion didn't count. I feel I'm being hit, hit, hit with all these words one right after another. I told her it's like you are hitting me with a hammer and I'm the rock that is getting broken down to rock dust and I get blown away with the wind.

I have to leave (second time I pack a suitcase). This time I pack only what I need for a few days. I leave certain items so it would seem as though I would have a place to come back to. Logical to me it was. I hate not knowing where I am anymore. I wish I could start my life all over with Brenda and Matthew.

Soon, I was in the psychotic state at my parents' home. A cold winter night. I felt I was into the future but not the future. I was trying to explain from the living room window to these E.T. space people that it wasn't nice or good for them to be killing innocent people for food for their planet. I explained to them it wasn't right and that we needed our heads, arms, and legs in order to live productive lives. I made gestures with my hand like an ax to my neck, arms, and legs. I explained by pointing and shaking my head—no! Then gesturing to them that I wanted to talk with one of them. The beings would not come into our house through the open sliding glass door. So I began with my little boy to try to explain to the E.T.s what sharing was. I picked up a golf ball and a small glass figurine. We proceeded to pass the two objects back and forth from my hand, then to my little boy's hand.

> **PN:** *From the mental health viewpoint, one can note that Craig is partly aware that he is psychotic.*

I know a few days ago we both had seen the E.T. video but this was the real thing. After our sharing explanation to E.T. I wanted to show my little boy that Daddy really knew E.T. was out there. So I placed the golf ball outside in the snow. I told him that E.T. would pick it up if he was really there. No luck, my boy wanted the golf ball back because he wanted to play with it and he didn't want E.T. to have it. So I asked him if it was OK to put the soccer ball out instead. "All right daddy," he said. We decided to go to bed and check it out in the morning. "The sun's up daddy, time to wake up." I cleaned up the house then looked outside and brought the partially deflated soccer ball in. It was cold and snowy so I washed it off in the kitchen sink where it resumed its full roundness.

I had a temporary job at an Automotive Factory. This job wasn't the cream of the crop but it might lead to a good wage with benefits. I met this black lady there who was a great inspiration to me and others. This person was highly regarded by me. One day while talking and walking with her I explained to her that I had seen the light. I told her it was a good feeling but it was also a little scary too. She told me she'd keep me in her prayers. This made me feel good inside. It seems as though when my schizophrenia comes on there is this network of people that come together around me. How true is this? Things happen around my unexplainable questions.

Friday before the weekend I was on this job that was one of the hardest jobs I'd ever done there. This job was supposed to be a one-man job. Me and this Mexican gentleman worked hard trying to keep up the supply for the others on the line—four hot molds to keep running while trying to keep everything organized. I jammed up one of the molds. I was sweating, thirsty, and wore a mask to keep the fumes and dust away from breathing. Later that evening I found out by ribbing from others on the line that the Mexican man I was working with was a police officer because I recognized his name.

On break with my working companion, I began thinking out loud to my foreman in the break room. Then I realized this other worker had heard me. My foreman jested to me to keep quiet or I could lose my head. Now Monday I was put on the same job but by myself. The lady I talked about earlier was at work with this very fancy black outfit on. She had this long leather coat with a hat on as if she was on her way to a church service. I then felt there was a very strong protection around me. These things really happened. Not hallucinating or a dream. Real, real, I tell you real. Do you believe me?

Next I'll tell you what happened. I went into this day dream state of mind trying to make sense of this, all in my mind. Thinking out loud again while working, I began to trip over myself by making mistakes. I had been thinking at work of the manuscript that I and Stuart had written together, the part about the KKK. While thinking about the manuscript, I thought my fellow workers were prisoners on a work release program, because I couldn't understand why anyone would take a job here as a career. I guess everyone has to provide shelter, food, and clothes for their families. While I was thinking this, the white man knew my thoughts and became very angry. His anger had been focused on me. At this point, he left his machine and charged over to where I was working to get me. Five kind men united to protect me from him. They tried to block my view of what was going on, but I caught a glimpse of two of them wrestling with him and dragging him away from me. These men, one oriental, two black, two white, I'd like to thank. I left work early without telling my foreman. My area would take lunch break early. It felt like the whole lunch break room had been vibrating as if the good over evil were confronting each other in a huge fight in the factory and also directly below me in the bathroom facilities. I had begun crying in the break room by myself as the second break people began filtering in. As I reached the bottom of the stairs and turned the corner, I then understood that my Vietnamese friend and a few other friends had taken care of the evil presence that was in the men's bathroom with Karate. I knew I had to do the right thing for everyone.

> **PN:** *Once again, note Craig's stark opposition of good and evil, without any awareness of shades of grey.*

I told one of the guys at my work station that I couldn't take it any more. So I left for home. I felt a world of relief as I drove away down the snow covered road. By leaving early, I made an unpredictable move on my part. The evil road drivers were not able to put together a defensive car or truck move on me.

Night time is when things begin to form into a new dimension. This is when I began following the cat around because I viewed him as my new protector. This part is sexual and personal, but I will reveal it in order to help others understand. I had fallen asleep in a comfortable chair. I am in the dream or sleep state of mind. Then I have a sexual hallucination with a woman that is the most incredible experience in my life. Later on I have another feeling that someone was filming this incredible lust between me and this woman. I felt that she wanted to have intercourse with me but I wouldn't let her because I didn't think it was right. (unexplainable differences)

The cat then lead me into this small room in the front of the house, where I positioned myself in front of this window to see out into the white winter night. I prayed to God and I was scared, so I asked God to send a messenger to explain or help me understand why all of this was happening to me. I felt that I was in the future in the time when Jesus Christ was on his way down to earth and that Gabriel, the angel, had been clearing the path for when the Saints come marching in. Gabriel was running the guillotine dressed with his armor, boots, and with a hammer and sword in hand. He would ask this very important question to each and every person one by one on earth. Do you believe in God? Do you believe in God? If they believed strongly, they would live. If not, then their life would end. There would stand two more angels who knew the good and bad of everyone on earth. If in question, Gabriel would refer to the two angels. I heard what sounded like hundreds of beings saying the Our Father. A bell would chime in between the prayers. I also heard vehicles pulling in and out of my folks' driveway as if looking for me to be questioned by Gabriel like all the others. But these small ghost people, whose shadows I could see, they had the red eyes like E.T., were protecting me and were extremely and intensely angry with me because I was going to take it upon myself to leave the small room.

PN: *One can note Craig's very florid delusions here. Gabriel the angel clears path for Jesus Christ, but Gabriel is described as "running the guillotine dressed with armor, boots, and with a hammer in his hands." He kills people who don't believe in God. Also, Craig shows the association of unrelated ideas. "Gabriel the angel had been clearing the path for when the Saints come marching in." These delusions seem quite consistent with those Craig experienced seven years earlier. Our research has shown consistency over time in the content of some of many schizophrenia patients' delusions (Harrow et al., 1995; Kaplan, Holtzman, Harrow, & Sands, 1993).*

With a gush of wind through the garage and into the house, this loud and powerful voice said, "Sit Down!" I obeyed the order. I sat down and looked out the window to see that the Christmas lights next door were out. The song of the little drummer boy was echoing through my head. Then I prayed for an angel or the Virgin Mary to be present to me, to relieve my fear. There was this shimmering shadow in which this beautiful voice called out, "here Kitty Kitty." The cat obeyed, jumped off my lap, and went over to be petted. I told the cat he was very lucky to know a person with such a beautiful beautiful voice.

Shortly after, I laid down for bed to sleep for the night. I don't know how all the pieces fit together in this complex puzzle in my head. I remember I made a telephone call to my brother Roger to tell him about my job situation. He told me to call the temporary service and explain to them that I had personal problems at home and that I would be at work today. I really didn't want to go to work, but I knew we needed the money and hopefully they might hire me. I didn't get much sleep last night so I took a nap.

After my nap I started getting ready for work. I was really scared to drive to work, but I had to do what was expected of me. I cleaned the snow off the car and warmed up the engine before starting out on my journey. This day there was good and bad drivers out on the road. When I reached the top of the driveway the car seemed to be lifted up high enough to see over the tall snow banks like on hydraulic shocks. The safe zone was now intact and ready to transport me to my job through the traffic. If there wasn't any job openings for a temporary service employee, that meant I'd end up pushing the broom or being sent home.

This gal slipped and fell while we waited for our job assignments. This guy started to laugh next to me. I think he realized I wasn't pleased with him for laughing at her. The foreman told me I'd be with Tom tonight.

Tom had me sweep up around some of the machines and stay out of sight of the office. I swept up the wet floor dry and put down the new on the oil that dripped from the machine. Tom looked real nervous and I felt the same. The thoughts going through my mind were that the enemy was closing in on me. Tom then told me that they didn't need me tonight and to check back in a month or so. I walked to the tool crib to return my broom. I told to the older lady in the tool crib that I was finished and might not be back. She had a half smile and her eyes looked a little tearful from my words and wished me luck. She said that she hoped she'd make it through the week end. I felt sorrow within me, with also the relief of leaving everything behind. I'm beginning to understand things all around me were changing to the degree of one hallucination after another.

I had the feeling that the road signs along side of the roads had been changed. I'm relating these kinds of trickery to the first time I was hospitalized in Cedar View. I knew I could outwit them in their games to confuse me. My turf, Lake City, and a different ball game this time around. I made it home, no thanks to the signs and autos. "I know what I know," Paul Simon, "Graceland." I can understand the angels in the architecture spinning around and around into infinity. Dad, you can call me Craig. Act 1 part 2 action, action I said. Puppets on strings. Straighten out latter. My younger brother spent a couple of nights with me. I was scared for him because I thought that he might be captured or killed on his journey to my folks house. I wasn't sure Alex was really Alex. The only reason he was allowed to enter was because he was my brother.

> **PN:** *One can note that Craig gives images of road signs being changed. He exhibits depersonalization—an image of movie or play— "Act 1 part 2 action," then "puppets on strings." His depersonalization is expressed in "feelings of being a puppet controlled by a script."*

There was a plastic surgeon outside who was able to put my brother back together if shot or dismembered. I wish I could please everyone but I can't. Neither can my wife. Breakdown of the family is on its way. Where do I fit in? I'm sorry for who I am? I hope God understands me for who I am? Sometimes I wish I could start over being a husband and a daddy. Alex brought over some beer and cigars. We watched some TV with our beer at hand. It was nice to spend some time with him. Why does my mind play tricks in thinking not to trust him but I do trust him right? Alex has been close because he has walked in shoes like mine. Roger hasn't quite fit the shoes. But all three of us have each walked in different paths that we all were inclined to take. We are brothers who might not understand each other's quest, but we are together as brothers. I felt Alex was fighting between being my brother or giving into the evil. I would sleep only a few hours then be awake and scared. Woke up Alex on the couch to talk to. To reinforce everything was all right. The next night I made Alex tell me that he believed in God before I let him come over to spend the night. He told me he did, so I let him come over to help me through another night.

Talked to Alex about my temporary job. Sometimes you need some personal days off from work in order to keep your sanity, which I found out. I called my sister-in-law to talk with me about my schizophrenic experiences and that I can't get any sleep the last three days or nights. I regarded my telephone conversation very highly with her because of my respect of her knowledge about me and where I'm coming from. Judy told me that the most important thing right now was sleep. I told her that I had been following the cat around and that Kitty Witty was comforting to me. She told me to take the kitty with me to snuggle with in bed. She also mentioned to me that an old wise man had told her that sleep was the most important thing right now. She also said that sometimes we do things that we just don't understand but that its all right. I thanked her and decided to take her advice, which made me feel better about myself. Days and time are hard to keep straight while writing.

> **PN:** *It is important to stress that Craig seems to have a trusting relation with his sister-in-law, Judy.*

My little boy, Matthew, was going to spend this night together with me. Also my wife was coming to town. I waited for Brenda in the small comfort room in the front of the house. While waiting for her to pull into the driveway, I was worrying because of the winter snow and the night time driving. I had this idea that these short E.T. people were outside waiting for my wife too. A female E.T. was going to be placed into my wife. They were pacing back and forth waiting for the arrival. I was thinking this was the way that they could conceive my sperm without disturbing my belief. I don't think they anticipated that my wife didn't really want to make love to me under the circumstances of being separated. Brenda and Matthew went to sleep in the living room. I tried but was not comfortable so I moved to the folks' bedroom. I listened to what Judy had told me that sleep was the most important thing for me right now. Oh to sleep through the night comfortably and peacefully again. It was hard for me to think that sleeping was the most important thing for me right now. I also was told that there might be things that I do that wouldn't make sense to me or others around me but that its all right to be different or to think I'm different in a good way.

I entered into a whole new concept of thought processing in which I'll explain. I made a choice in my mind to populate the E.T. generation, because I thought it would mean a lot to our future. Then I positioned myself in bed to face the east. Also to see down the lighted hallway. I felt as though I had traveled into a futuristic state of mind. I felt that there was only a select few that had made it as far as I have into this futuristic mode of thinking. The select few were made up of people from every race and religion. I feel that I have made it to an organization of people who think of things in an open point of view like mine. At this point, I realized that I might die before my time. So I sent out this beacon of distress signals in order to bring me back to where I had been before my travels. Judy has been as far and farther than I into the future. So I had to leave her clues in order for her to find me. I had to be very careful because it had become a very complex puzzle. One wrong clue or slip up it could end our lives and existence forever on earth as we know it today.

> **PN:** *Craig is both aware and not aware of being ill. He says he is aware of "a new concept of thought processing." Craig feels he is able to "send out beacons of distress signals."*

Judy made it as far as the doorway to the garage. But she couldn't make it into the house. Her next choice happened to be the window to the bedroom in which I lay in wait. A cold winter breeze blew gently, as a snake slithered past the venetian blinds and dropped to the floor. In a faint whisper I could hear some relaxing words from Judy as she entered into the house. Surprise, surprise I felt foolish. It had all been a joke to tell me that I had become one of the few that had made it into the elite organization of the wise.

I awoke to this orange glow of smoke creeping down the hallway. As I passed from the hallway into the living room the whole floor was red as hot charcoal from a grill. As I lay my pillow down on the love seat to try to sleep, a fire engulfed the deck and then disappeared. Then a single tree became like torch—a reminder of the burning bush from the Bible. The fireplace in the living room had become two fireplaces. Which I then began figuring out that the clues had been placed there in order for me to find out that I had been chosen to take over when my father passes away.

> **PN:** *We again can note the fusing of religious and psychotic themes. Craig gives a Biblical image of the Burning Bush, but it becomes distorted into various images. Craig feels a clue has been given for him to replace his father when his father dies. Note that this is not an Oedipal but a Biblical image. This involves not competition with his father, but succession of him (Kaplan, 1990).*

My uncle showed up the next day to go out to lunch with us. Alex also showed up to see how things were going with me. Numbers played a big part in controlling a peaceful and calm atmosphere. One-on-one or one-on-two discussion with me was bearable, but more people than this was difficult for me to handle. I would have to leave the room if there was more people than I could handle. Three like Brenda, Matthew, and my uncle I could just handle, but when Alex entered, it threw off my balance of people I could handle around me at this time. I know I was acting different, but I couldn't help it. I was trying to tell everyone I was OK and just needed something to help me sleep at night.

> **PN:** *Note that Craig shows partial awareness of his illness. For example, in the next passage Craig shows awareness that he might obsessively talk "about things in the room over and over again."*

It was suggested to me to try and get something to help me through the weekend. I tried my doctors office, but he wasn't able to prescribe any psychiatric medication. I didn't have a regular psychiatrist or doctor since I hadn't needed any medications in the last five years. I then decided to go down to the hospital to see if there was anything they could do to help me get through the nights with some sleep. Before I left the house, I left my family members with instructions not to leave the house until they could see my car go by the house down the road. This was something I had to do on my own because I didn't want any harm to come to any of my family.

I entered the hospital and made my way down to the emergency room. They had taken down some information on me. They had me wait in a small room for someone to come and talk to me. A nurse come in to take a few vital signs. I then began my process of my stay in a wheelchair in the emergency room. A policeman sat down next to me. I told this guy that everything was alright but strange things always happen around me and that I was glad he was here. The fire alarm began going off around us, but this was OK because we heard over the intercom that we'd be having a fire alarm test.

Things just happen for no reason at all around me. I also explained to him that when I talk to him I might start talking about things in the room over and over again but not to worry. It's just something I do. A young man came up to me and explained to me that he was here to talk to me. He asked if it would be OK to talk to me in the small waiting room. I went over my same explanation of having to talk about things in the room over and over again. I also explained to him that it was easier for me to talk on a one-to-one basis. After my talk with this nice gentleman, I was lead to the ward 2 North where my stay would prevail.

My first two days I felt that I was on this spaceship because it seemed as though the floor was vibrating and moving. I felt as though this E.T. being had entered my body. This doctor had come into the ward to talk to me. My mind figured out the reason this doctor was so heavy was because he was wearing a space suit. And he had me enter this room which seemed as if it was air pressurized. I was to be presented with this test—*Millon Clinical Multiaxial Inventory-II*—to be completed by me. I was to fill out one of these tests three times during my stay at the hospital.

> **PN:** *Note Craig's feelings of boundary violation. He feels that this "E.T. being had entered my body."*

I was confined to this lock-up area with one other patient. Sam was this elderly man who was confined to a wheel chair. This man was able to channel evil people from my earlier hospitalization in 1978 to the room that we occupied. We each were split 50/50 vs. evil and good. He tried very hard to break me down and catch me off guard. Sam had relatives who would come and visit just about every day. I felt the most uncomfortable with him and his visitors. I came to believe Sam had been informing them that I was Craig. Everyone on the staff had been informing people that I was a she or lady because my voice seems to change tones at times. This was to throw any would-be assailants off my trail. A larger amount of visitors were visiting Sam. I began to hear talk of who was going to be the one to do the job with the gun they managed to get into the room. I had been conveying my thoughts of pure fright.

> **PN:** *Note that Craig gives an image of he and his roommate "split 50/50 vs. evil and good." Does this mean each of them is split 50/50 between good and evil? This marks an advance over previous splitting of good versus evil (that one person is entirely evil and the other entirely good) so typical of borderline patients.*

I reached across the desk to the nurse, and she held my hand to realize she was scared too. I never experienced anything like this fast rush that came up to me grabbed my out-stretched arm and did a flip around and then vanished to the back of the ward. I was beginning to relax more and more with these E.T. type of encounters. Back to gun play. All these visitors and just the two of us. What were they waiting for? My lady friend got up, went over to the table, and told them that this wasn't allowed on the ward. I understood it to be the gun that was to end my life. I couldn't believe she actually did what she did.

> **PN:** *Note the strange suicidal image of gun play. "The gun that was to end my life." Craig externalizes the blame on the lady friend, "I couldn't believe she actually did what she did."*

I'll explain some of the people who worked around me and how this came to be. The weather outside was very bad to try and drive around in. There had been so many car accidents around that the workers had an over abundant supply of body parts to keep them covered in human skin. E.T. people were the workers. They could only wear the skins for a certain amount of time before they needed to change. Some of the workers needed to just change an arm, and other legs or hands. Full body change lasted longer than just parts. I had begun to scale down the workers I was going to put my trust in. The one person, Pat, seemed to be the key person out of everyone who held the strongest protection organization leader to me. Even though she hadn't worked closely with me, I always knew her presence was around.

> **PN:** *Note Craig's bizarre image of workers with an overabundant supply of body parts to keep them covered in human skin.*

One day, I decided to read to myself from the large print *Readers Digest.* Over a period of time, I began testing the workers one by one. Can you believe it: a schizophrenic quizzing the psychiatric workers on the ward about schizophrenia? This *Readers Digest* was one of the best tests for the so-called white supremacist. Laughter is the best medicine. I went on reading out loud to see their reactions. I told them that it was lucky I found this book because I was curing myself with laughter as I laughed and laughed to their uncomfortable anger brewing inside of them. The book made references to colors, vegetables, and fruit. The only comeback they had was to medicate me.

The medications I encountered at this point hit me like a ton of bricks. Strongest dose I've ever encountered on the ward. I felt as though I was sinking deeper and deeper into the floor. It was as if I had sunk about two and a half feet where my knees were just about to the point I could walk on them without the rest of my legs. Pills do help only if given with care. Eyes would blur because of medications. End of reading the *Digest* book tonight.

I had to have a code word that only my relatives or friends would know in order for them to visit or talk to me on the phone while I was in the lock-up section. I had chosen my middle name, Joseph, because I like it. My Uncle Don visited me in lock-up. I told him I was doing OK and decided to show him some of my drawings because I was very proud of the way I had incorporated color into them now, rather than just black and white. It sure is nice to have family who care about you. Roger and Judy also visited me in lock-up. They asked if I needed anything and brought back a small supply to help me through my stay. My wife and boy also came to visit too. I gave her a picture for a Valentine's Day so she and Matthew could have something beautiful to look at to remember Daddy by.

The day I left lock-up felt very good to me, but my behavior changed slightly. I would play the clothes game. It also dealt with the colors I wore. I'd change a few times a day to confuse anyone who might be after me to kill or hurt me. The cleaning lady was their contact with Sam or others. She stuck her tongue out at me. It had turned black on the tip. I thought I could trust. Because of the episode with the gun. The tip of her tongue was black too.

> **PN:** *Again note Craig's paranoid tendencies. He gives an image of the "clothes game." Craig says he changes clothes and colors to confuse anyone who might be trying to kill him.*

Another one of the workers who loved opera and talked like Zsa Zsa Gabor I felt was leading a group to me to kill me. They were on the floor below me and proceeded with the help from the little drummer boy's music. My whole room would vibrate and shake during the march through the rooms and halls killing people. The noise would dissipate with time. I got myself into the system or routine to satisfy them and to prove I was OK. I felt there were cameras everywhere to watch my every move. Even in the shower stalls. It seemed they used these videotapes for their own entertainment. They would splice people in and out of the tapes to protect themselves from all the killing that went on in the shower stalls. (It also seemed to me while in lock-up workers would lose a finger by this small cutting device to keep silence of my whereabouts. Also while in lock-up the person at the desk could communicate with others with this small clicking device like a Morse code transmitter.)

Before I got there, there was a lot more openness about sex between workers and patients. Even the administrator proved that to be a fact. Is my mind keeping up with my thoughts I'm processing? Could this be a soap opera thing I may be picking up in my mind. My favorite place to be is the fishbowl room. I guess because of all the windows and it made me feel secure. Little Korea was always there too with her cameras photographing me the schizophrenic during a hospital stay. It was nice to have someone else around trying to understand and document the events of a schizophrenic. I felt it would help others understand the real human behind the hidden schizophrenic mask that may have never before been revealed before. If this is a true statement I hope it does help? From my fishbowl room, I could peer out into the real world. One thing was that I could control the weather in this room by an open window into the cold winter night. I left this window alone to the outside because a bird had made a nest between the open window and the stationary one. Every once in a while this little bird would come to visit me. Where upon I could enjoy the beautiful music of nature. Color has now been a big part of me to present beautiful places of peace and harmony through naturalistic realism. I have always told people that my artwork was my escape from reality, but what is reality anymore?

> **PN:** *Craig gives an image of being schizophrenic. "From my fish-bowl, I could peer out onto the real world." Over the last few pages, he also has given a picture of some of the terrifying images he experienced of threats to kill or mutilate him. This theme too is consistent with that experienced in his earlier, psychotic episodes.*

I would watch it snow from my observatory window with the faint sound of a circus marching band making its way down the street to the front door of the hospital. The leader of the band was none other than my little boy Matthew Joseph Geiser who was coming on into the hospital to cheer up his daddy. What more could a father ask for. I love that little guy. I want to tell everyone that the food was the best I've ever had from a hospital facility before.

I don't think I mentioned this before but I have new freedoms, like going for a walk with staff to have a cigarette. Oh to smoke again, what a relief that is. The nicotine patches helped but to inhale again that was the ultimate desire. I put up with the snow melting and the ice covered sidewalks to smoke my cigarettes. I was nervous on these sidewalks because the worker who was with me I thought was trying to contact people along our route to do me in. I caught the lady worker before she fell to the ground. She wasn't prepared for the icy puddle jumping we all had to do while we had our smoke. Later on I gained the right to go out on my own on a time limited basis. There was a variety of classes I agreed upon to take for a while.

My relatives met with me and my therapist to decide how things were going to be for me on an outpatient basis. Things were going OK for me with the classes but by the end of the first week I decided I wasn't benefiting from the hospital atmosphere. So the whole next week I met only with my therapist once that week. I decided to try meeting for the classes one more time if my insurance would allow me to reenter as an outpatient again. So this week went real good until Friday.

I had a difficult time being in large groups of people. So I decided to discontinue the hospital for a second time. I felt discouraged and all by myself. I would walk to the hospital and back to my folks house while attending the outpatient program. On my walks I had this funny feeling I was being followed by many different vehicles who were out on the roads to protect me by surveillance. One time on my last walk home I felt as though I had this friend that was by my side as I walked home. I knew there was this special presence there because as we walked some stones were being kicked up along side of me.

> **PN:** *Note that Craig again seems aware of his illness. He reports a difficult time being in large groups of people. He decided to discontinue the hospital again. Craig feels he was being followed by many vehicles who were trying to protect him.*

While at my parents home one day I had decided I had to get out of the house for a while. I started out on a hike that would take me on this five-mile trek. It was lightly snowing out as I preceded to a place I had to check out for myself. As I walked, the snow and wind would have chilled anyone to the bone but I had my mind set that I had to talk to the minister of this church. I grabbed up this white shoe I had found on my journey because I thought this would be my protection from any evil persons who would want to kill me. Snow had now covered me from head to toe. I tried one door on the church locked. I kept trying until I found a door that would swing open. I proceeded through these halls till I had come to these people of whom I had asked to talk to the minister. This was the faith of the church of which this lady from the factory had belonged to. I wanted to see the ministers of whom she enlisted her faith with. It just so happened to be a gentleman I went to high school with. I wasn't sure if this was the place I could find help for my schizophrenia, but I had to try something because this sickness seems to be taking over my life and I just wanted to be normal again. They told me they could help but I would have to follow some strict rules. I wasn't sure, but they helped me get some prayers and the laying of the hands on my head. They were very kind people and offered me a ride home which I had accepted thankfully. They offered me rides back and forth to their church in which I had accepted.

> **PN:** *Again note the merger of religious and psychotic themes. Craig picks up a white shoe that would be his protection from people who want to kill him. Craig goes to church to attempt to find help for his schizophrenia.*

After thinking it over for a while, I made a phone call to the minister the day before church to decline the offer that was made to me. I then decided to go to this church down the road a little ways from my folks house. Some friends of mine were members there, and I thought it might be good for me and Matthew to attend. Matthew enjoyed it because he got to play with all kinds of kids, but I didn't feel comfortable there. I wish I could, but right now I don't. Matthew sure had fun there. Still have trouble being around large groups of people. Marriage counselors didn't work. Brenda and I are getting a divorce.

CRAIG'S DRAWINGS

My drawings have helped me relax, and they give me an opportunity to leave the real world and go into fantasy and make believe—in a constructive fashion. I do not really know how to explain my drawings. I never know how my drawings are going to turn out. I just pick up my pen and guide it on the paper and when I set it down, my drawings are satisfying to me and I hope more people will enjoy them. Someone told me she had found them interesting, that they are of people or creatures, and that the focal point of them is often the eyes. They made her think of the idea that the eyes are the window of the soul.

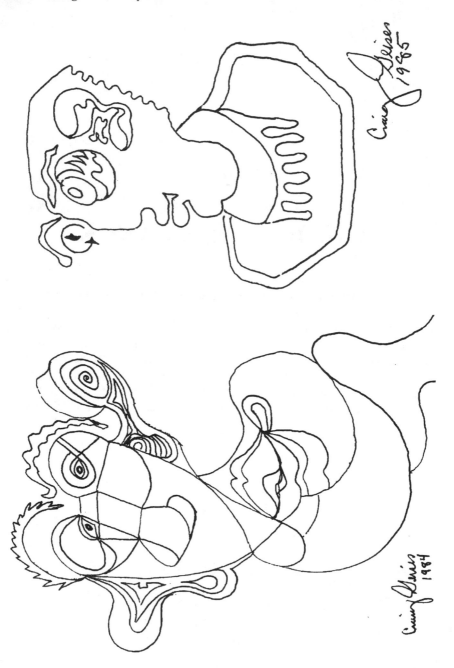

Drawings 1 (top) and 2 (bottom).

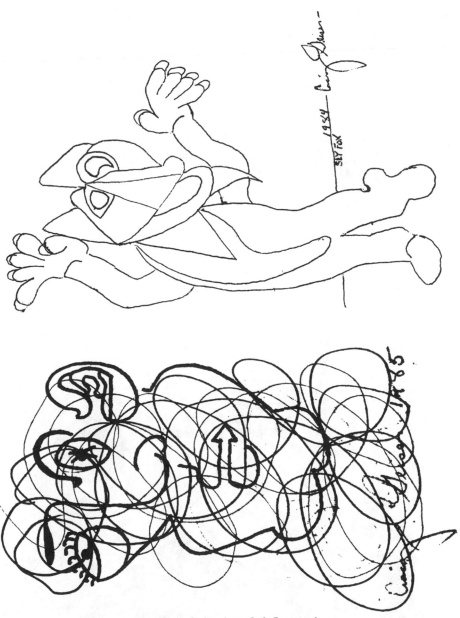

Drawings 3 (top) and 4 (bottom).

PN: *It is important to note the asymmetry in the eyes indicating perhaps a conflicting personality or perhaps a discrepancy between a distorted and realistic perception of the world. This theme reappears in many of Craig's drawings.*

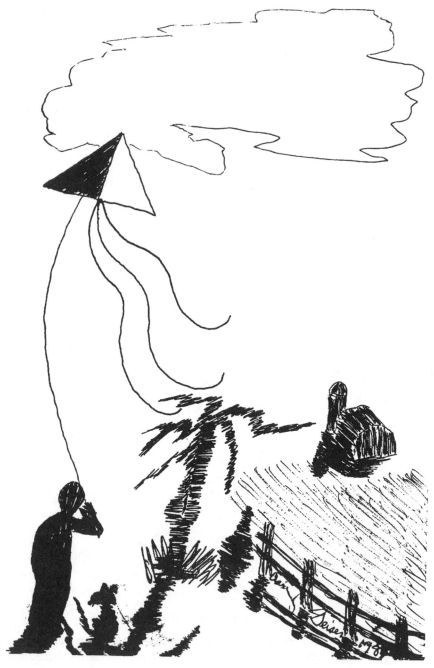

Drawing 5.

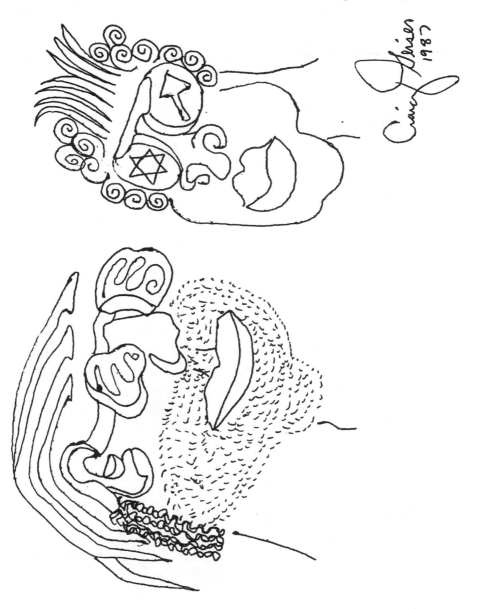

Drawing 6.

PN: *Notice the inappropriate placement of the Star of David in the left eye. This theme reappears in later drawings. Again notice the asymmetry in the eyes.*

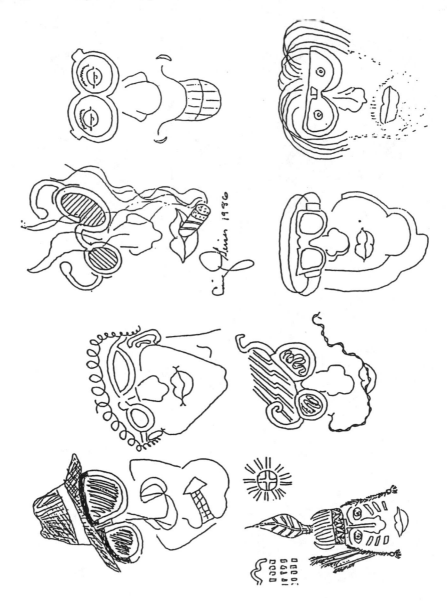

Drawing 7.

PN: *Note the paranoid representation of different ethnic types, often portrayed as sinister types. Each of these figures wears glasses that cannot be seen into. This may represent Craig's sense that the world is watching him but cannot be watched in return.*

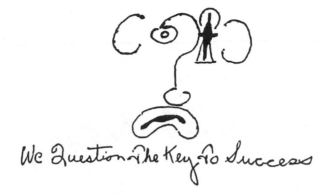

We Question The Key To Success

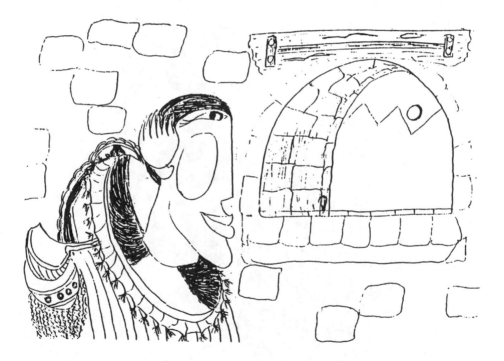

Drawing 8.

PN: *Note the Cyclops-like portrayal of a figure with one eye in the middle of his forehead instead of two in the bottom half of Drawing 8. We will see this portrayal in several other drawings.*

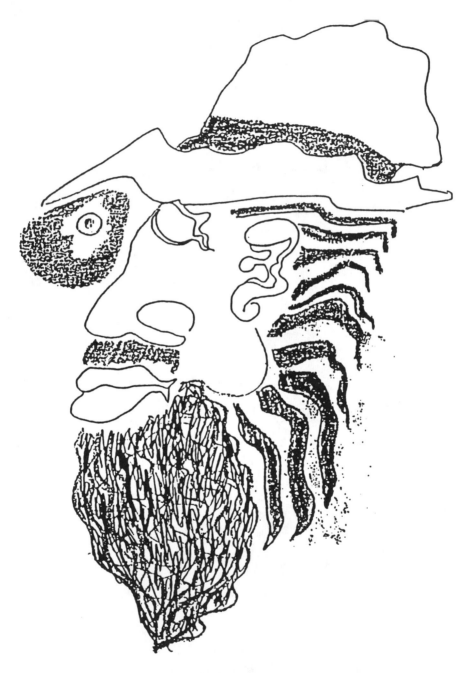

Drawing 9.

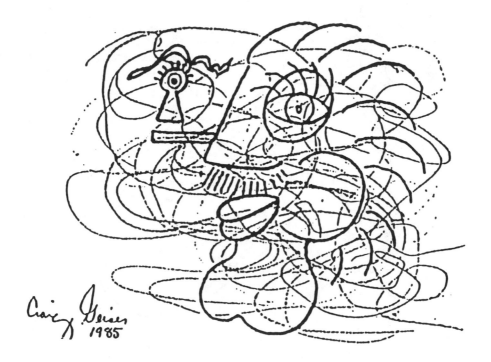

Drawing 10.

PN: *Again, notice the asymmetry of the eyes in Drawing 9 and the single eye in Drawing 10.*

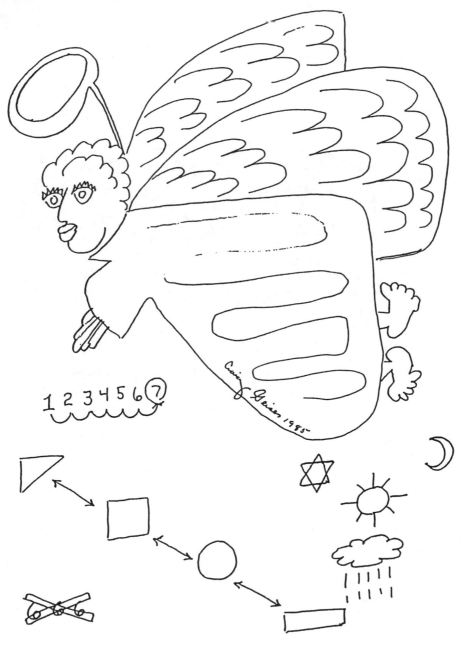

Drawing 11.

PN: *Again, see the Star of David below the flying angelic figure.*

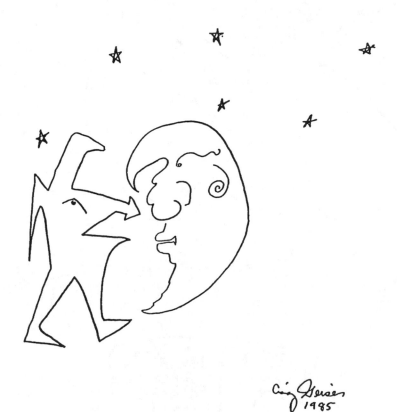

Drawing 12.

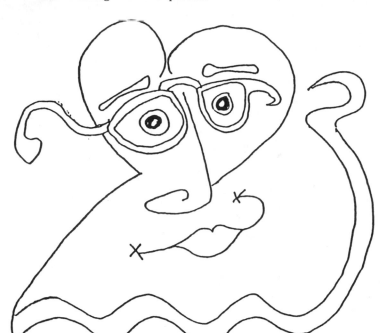

your THE HeArT of My LiFE Craig Greiser 1985

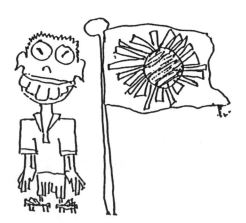

Drawings 13 (top) and 14 (bottom).

PN: *In Drawing 14, note Craig's portrayal of Asian faces.*

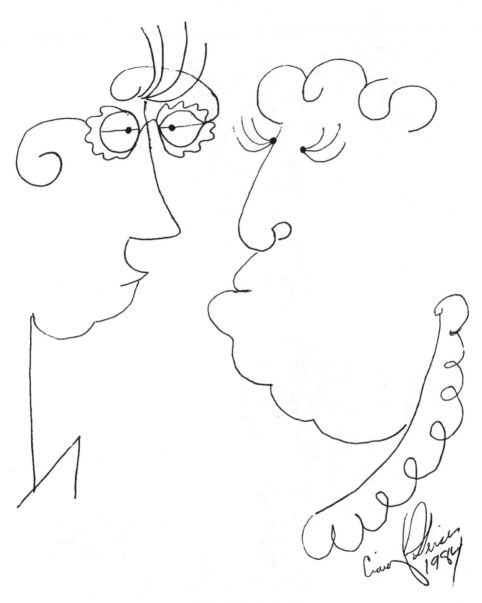

Drawing 15.

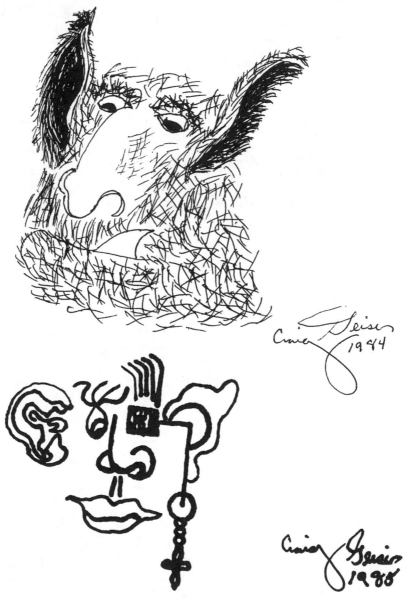

Drawings 16 (top) and 17 (bottom).

PN: *Notice the asymmetry of the eyes in Drawing 17 and the reversal of the figure and ground of the two eyes. In the left eye, the pupil is in the foreground, and in the right eye, the pupil seems to recede and the white comes forward.*

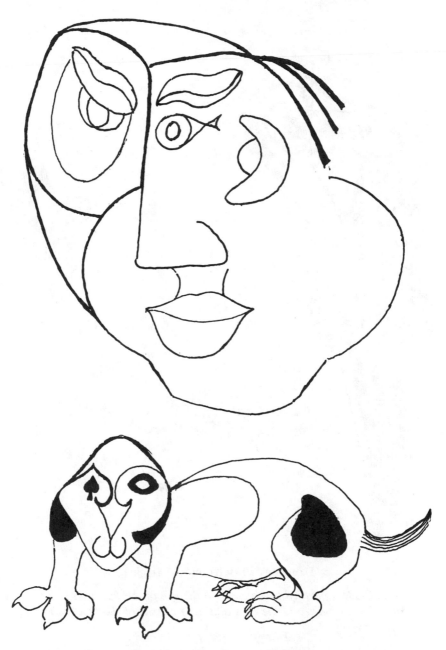

Drawings 18 (top) and 19 (bottom).

PN: *Again, note the asymmetry of the eyes in Drawings 18 and 19.*

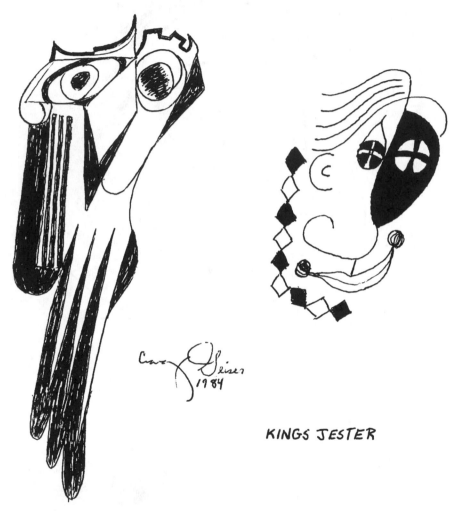

KINGS JESTER

Drawings 20 (left) and 21 (right).

PN: *Note Craig's portrayal of a cross in the eye of the figure in Drawing 21. Note also the asymmetry of the eyes and the reversal of the black-white figure found in Drawing 21.*

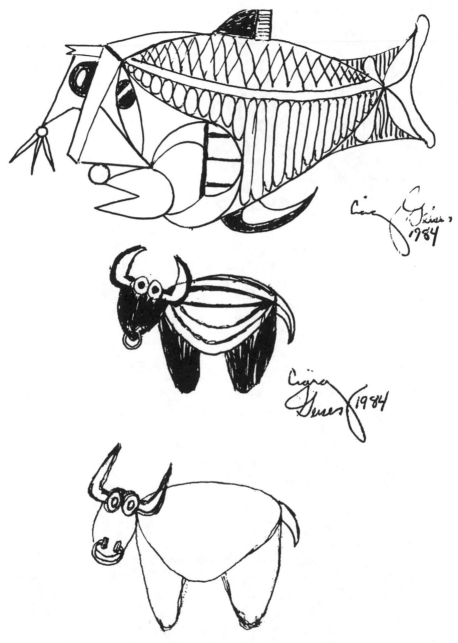

Drawings 22 (top) and 23 (bottom).

PN: *Notice the black-white reversal figure ground for Drawing 23.*

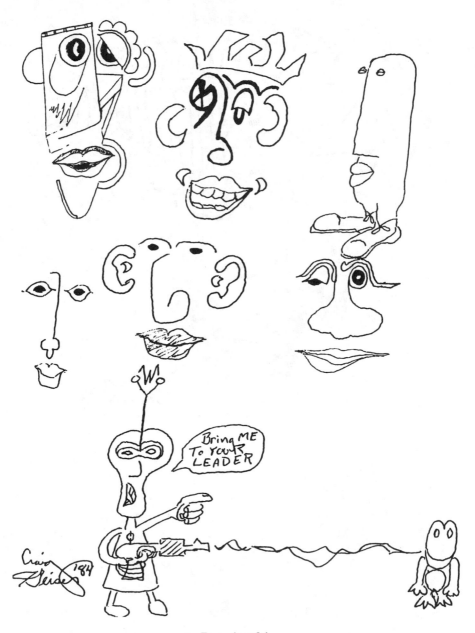

Drawing 24.

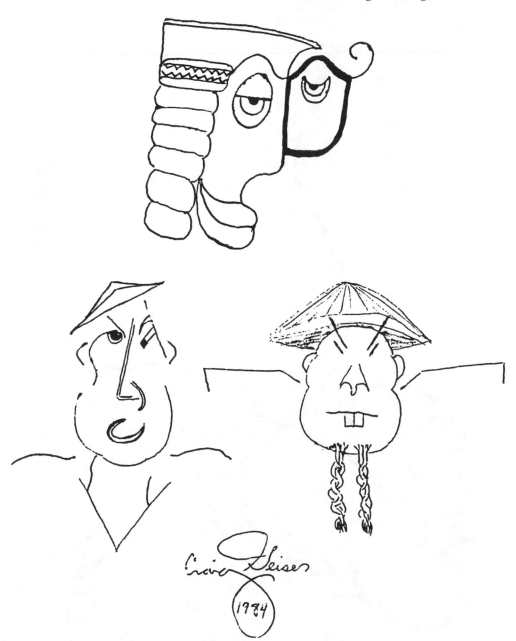

Drawings 25 (top) and 26 (bottom).

PN: *Again, note the portrayal of the Asian faces in Drawing 26.*

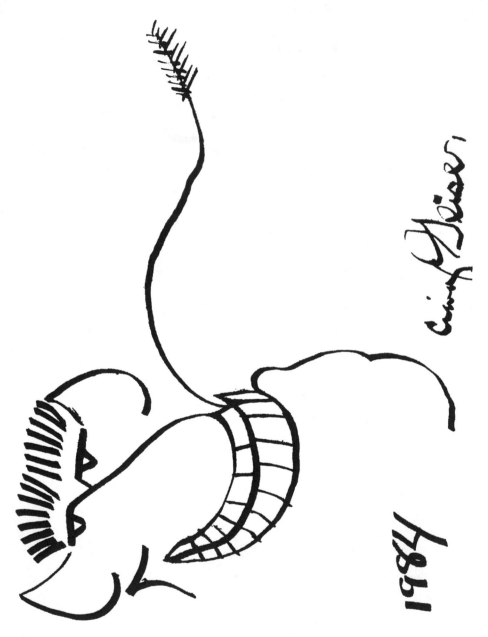

Drawing 27.

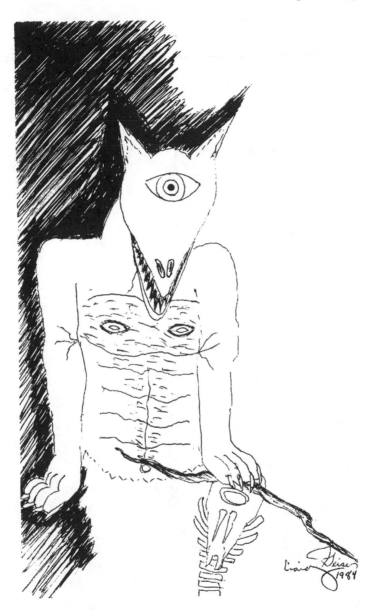

Drawing 28.

PN: *Note again the reappearance of the one-eyed Cyclops in the face of the figure represented above, but the suggestion of eyes in place of nipples on the chest.*

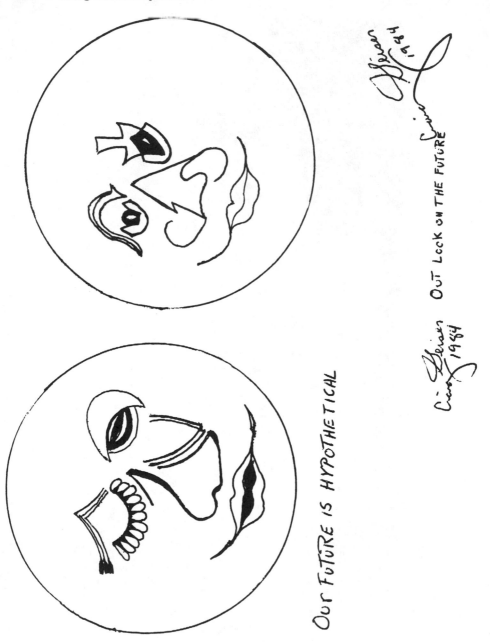

Drawings 29 (top) and 30 (bottom).

PN: *Again, note the full asymmetry of the eyes in the two drawings.*

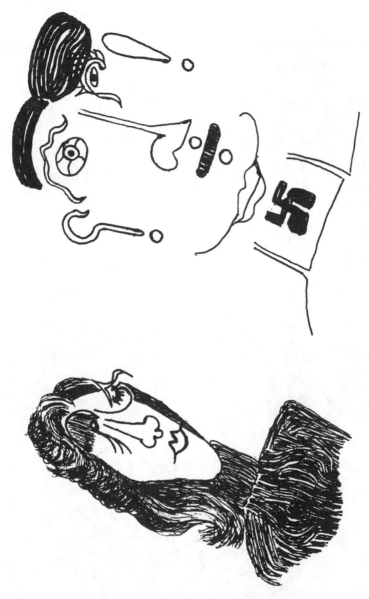

Drawings 31 (top) and 32 (bottom).

PN: *Note here the drawing of a Hitler-like figure with a swastika on his chest. Note also that his eyes are represented by punctuation marks, his right ear being a reversed question mark, and his left ear being an exclamation mark. Again, note the asymmetry in both figures' eyes.*

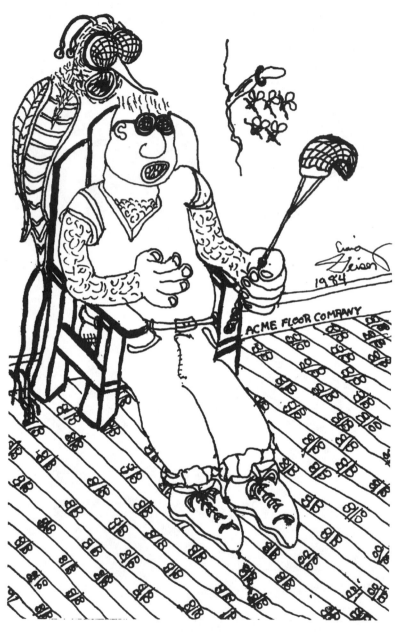

Drawing 33.

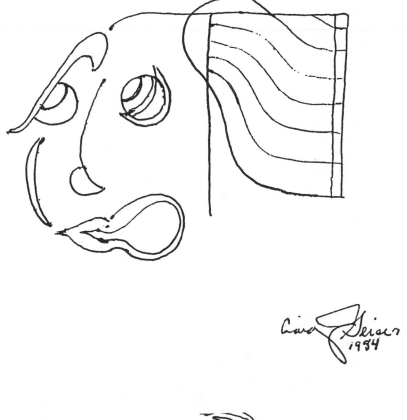

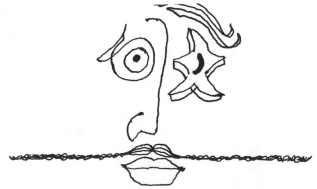

Drawings 34 (top) and 35 (bottom).

PN: *Note the image of fish and water in Drawing 35. Notice also the asymmetry of the eyes.*

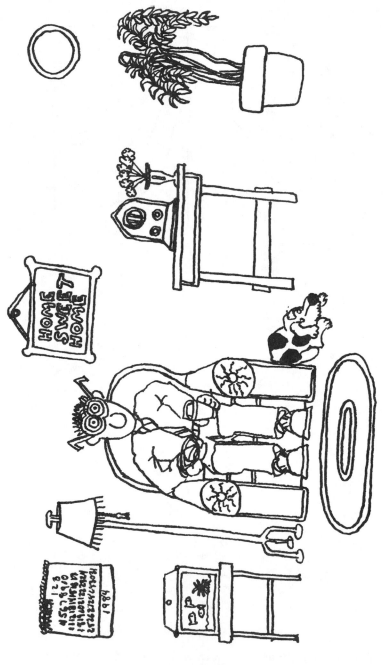

Drawing 36.

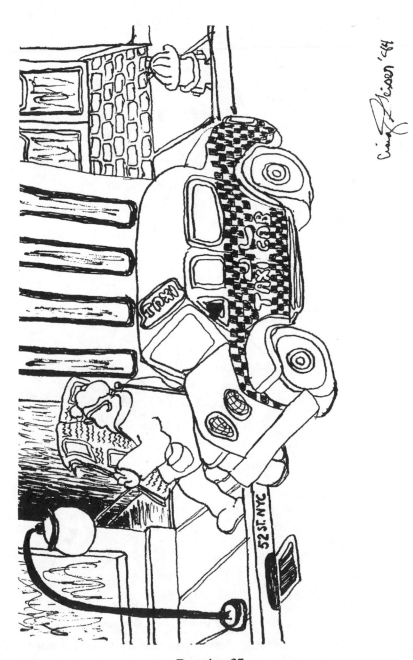

Drawing 37.

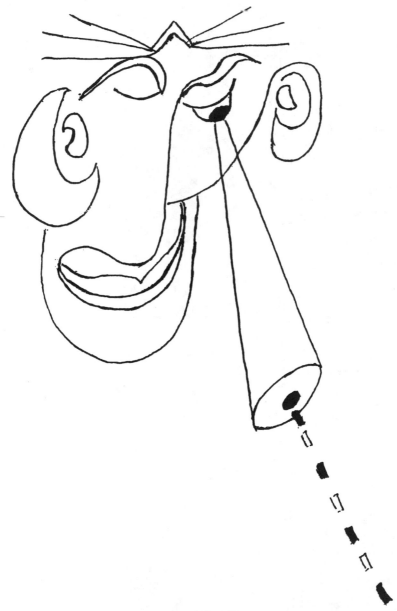

Drawing 38.

PN: *It is important to note Craig's extension of an eye into a telescope. This again suggests a paranoid preoccupation. The world is watching him through a telescope.*

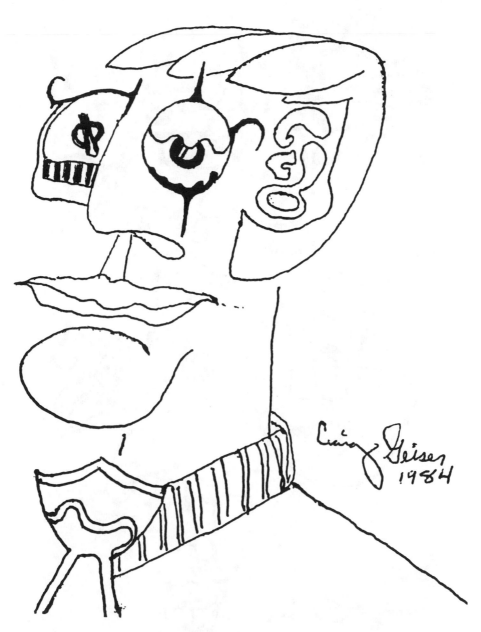

Drawing 39.

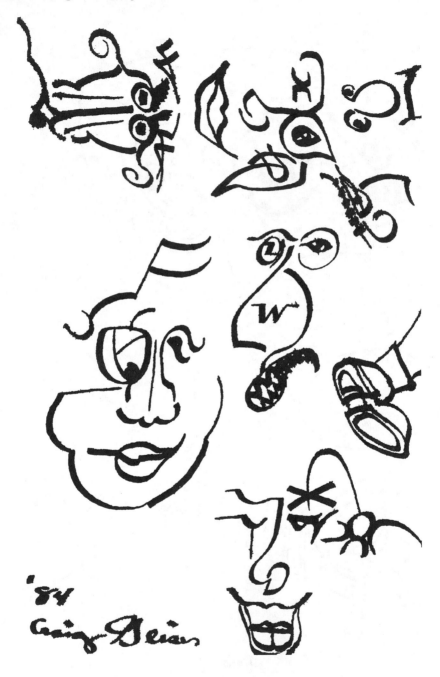

Drawing 40.

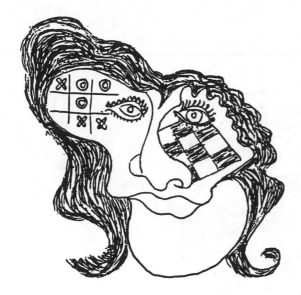

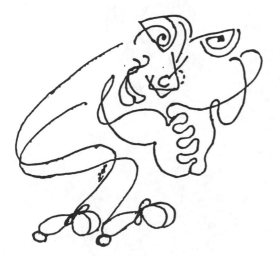

Drawings 41 (top) and 42 (bottom).

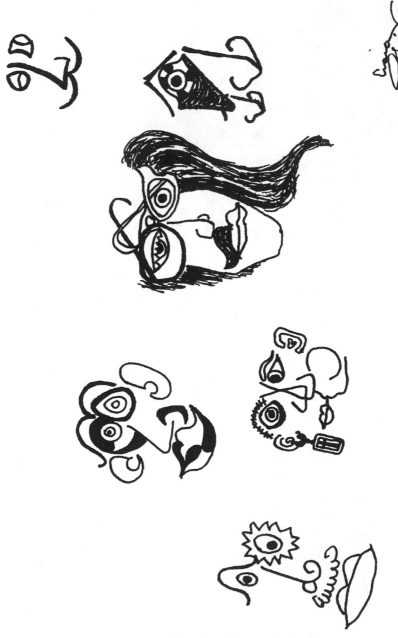

Drawing 43.

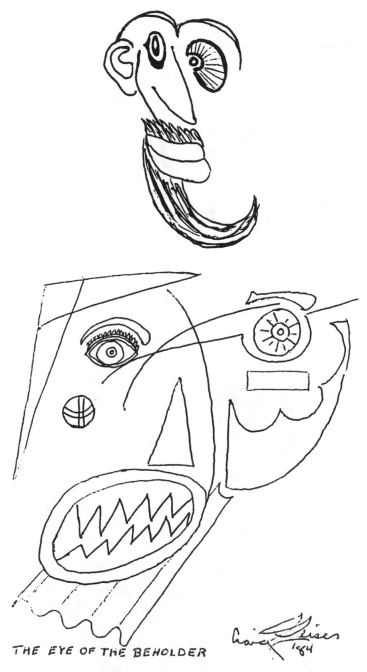

THE EYE OF THE BEHOLDER

Drawings 44 (top) and 45 (bottom).

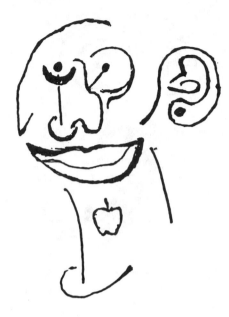

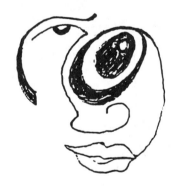

Drawings 46 (top) and 47 (bottom).

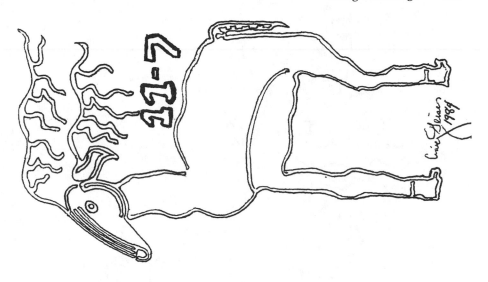

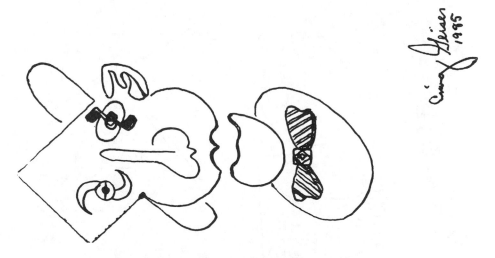

Drawings 48 (top) and 49 (bottom).

PN: *Note in Drawing 49 the black-white reversal of the two eyes. The one on the left eye suggests a part of a Communist side, and the one on the right suggests part of a Nazi swastika.*

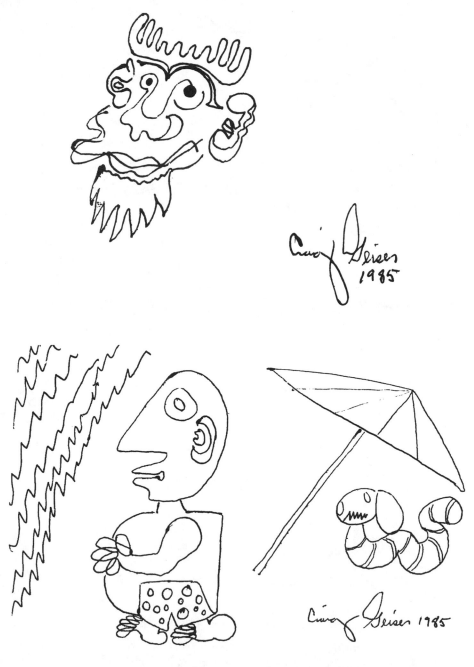

Drawings 50 (top) and 51 (bottom).

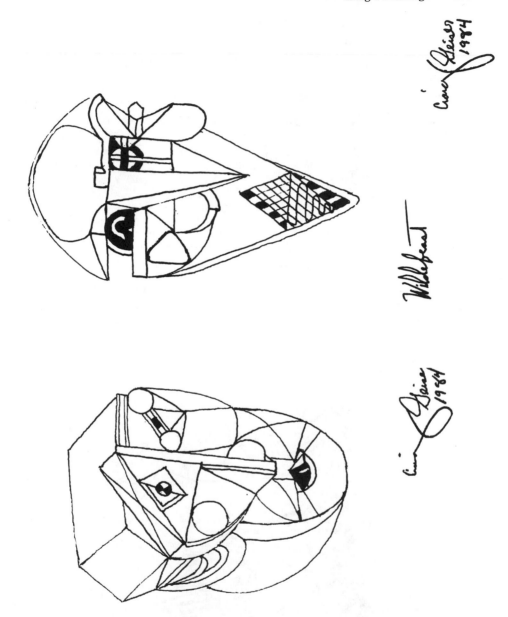

Drawings 52 (top) and 53 (bottom).

PN: *Again note the asymmetry of the eyes. Note Craig's striking geometric forms in his creation of the faces. Again note Craig's employment of a cross in the right eye in Drawing 52.*

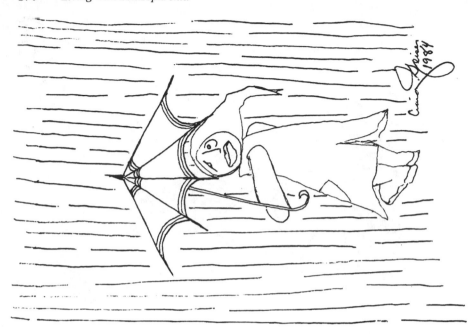

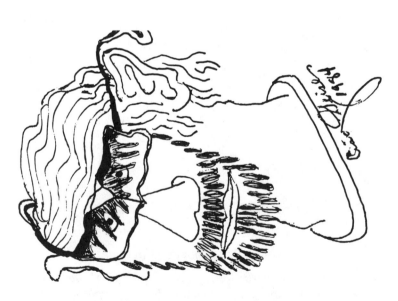

Drawings 54 (top) and 55 (bottom).

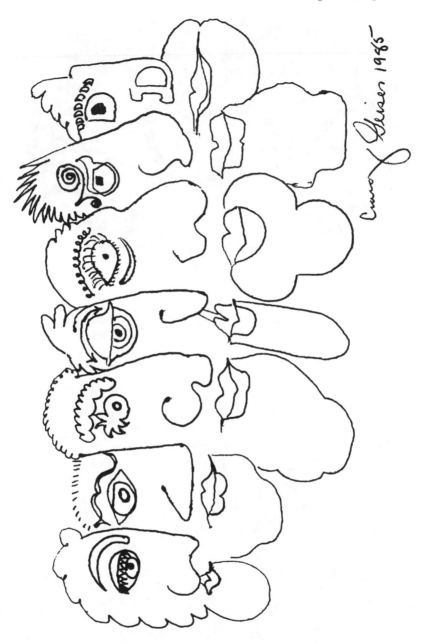

Drawing 56.

PN: *Note the image of the one eye of multiple figures in Drawing 56.*

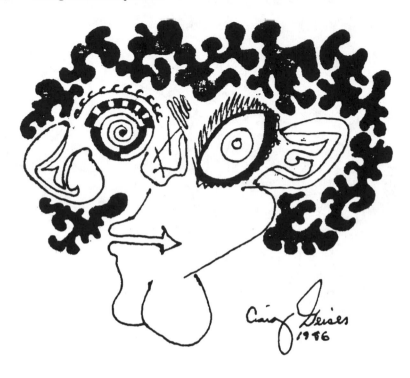

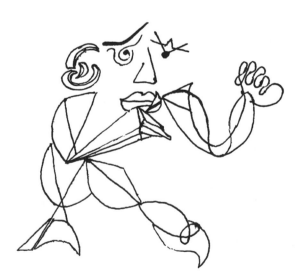

Drawings 57 (top) and 58 (bottom).

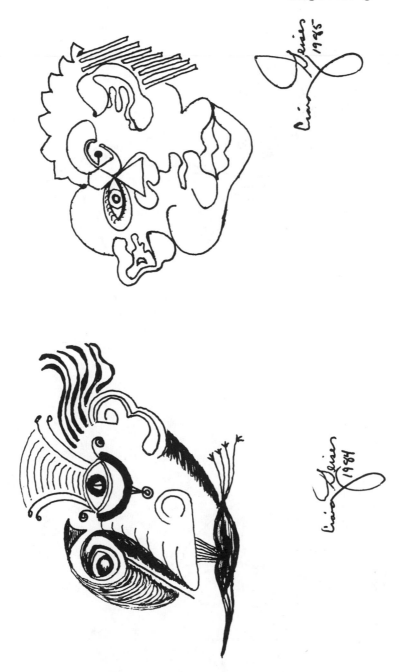

Drawings 59 (top) and 60 (bottom).

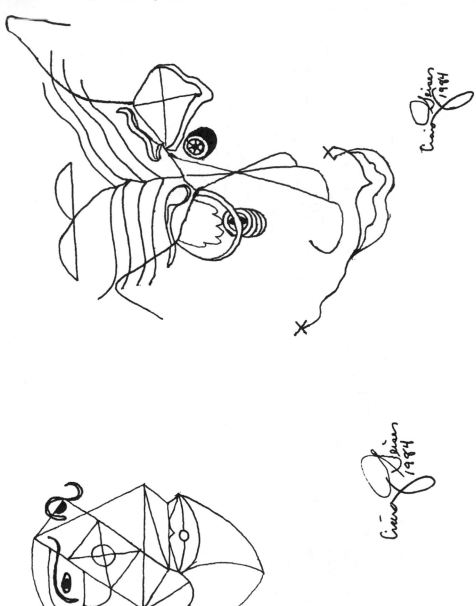

Drawings 61 (top) and 62 (bottom).

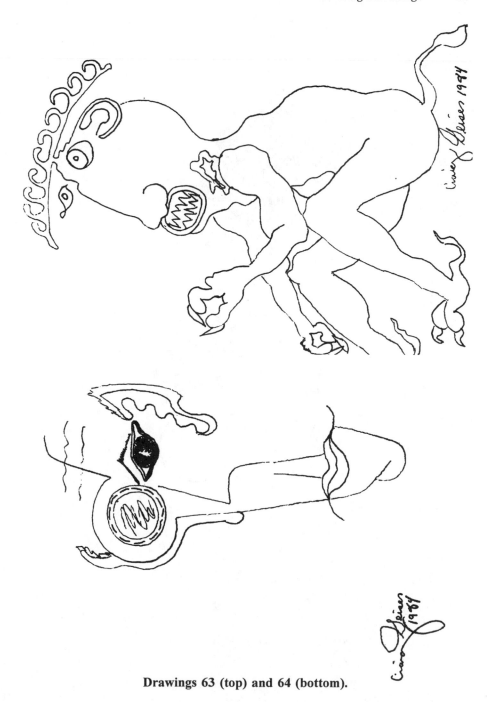

Drawings 63 (top) and 64 (bottom).

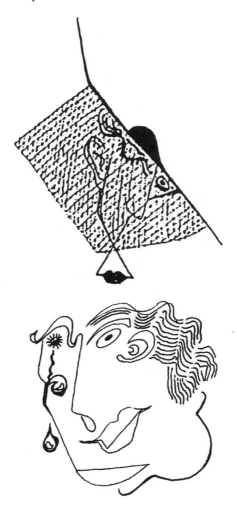

Drawings 65 (top) and 66 (bottom).

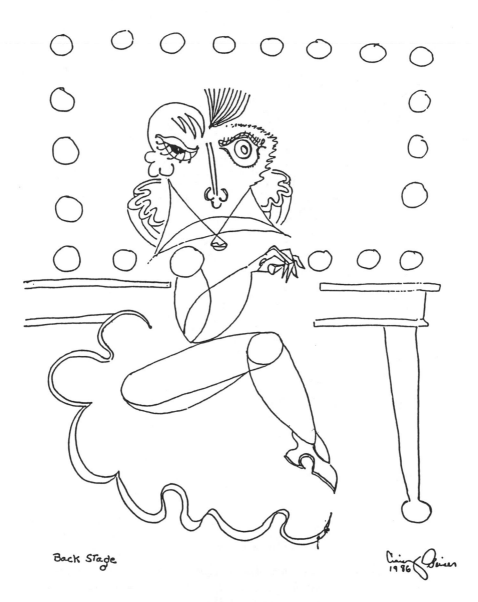

Back Stage

1986

Drawing 67.

PN: *Note the asymmetry in the eyes and the reversal of the black-white to foreground in the two eyes.*

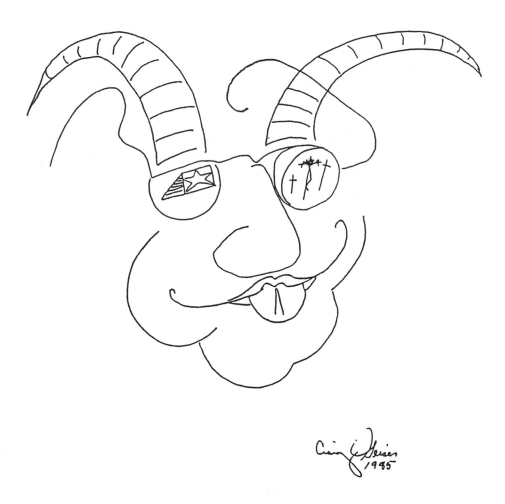

Drawing 68.

PN: *Note the asymmetrical content within the two eyes—an American Star on the left and three crosses on the right with a body draped on the middle cross. This represents a New Testament theme of Jesus being brought on the cross to Pontius Pilot flanked by two other Jewish prisoners, also on crosses.*

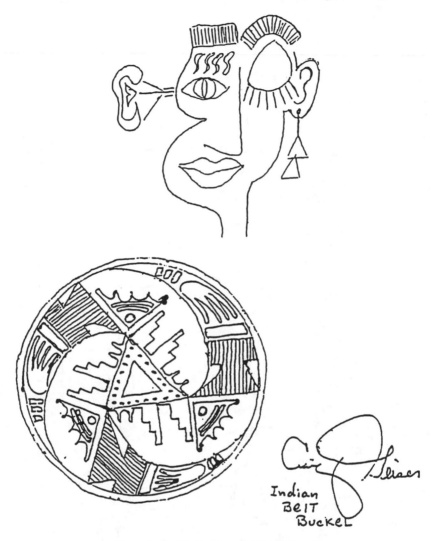

Drawings 69 (top) and 70 (bottom).

PN: *In Drawing 69, note the asymmetry of the eyes and the detached ear. Craig describes Drawing 70 as follows: "I had this belt with a belt buckle made by an Indian in New Mexico. this belt buckle symbolized safety for me in my stay in the hospital. I felt no harm would come to me while I wore it. I also left it visible to me on my nightstand next to my bed at night. I thought several times the belt buckle saved me from whatever was going on. My belt buckle seemed as though it was wearing thinner, using up its strength a little at a time in helping me."*

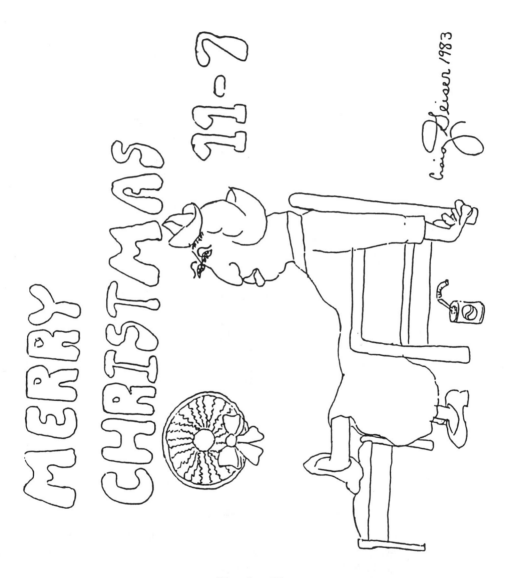

Drawing 71.

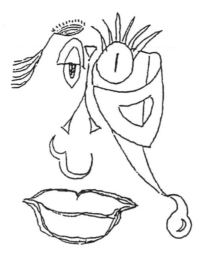

DAYS GONE BYE WITH NOTHING ACCOMPIJSHED

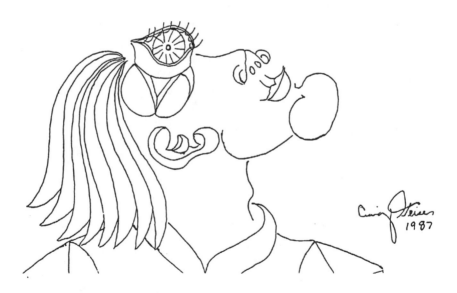

Drawings 72 (top) and 73 (bottom).

PN: *Note again the Cyclops image of one eye emerging from the socket in a very marked fashion. From a mental health perspective, such emphasis on the eyes indicates paranoia. The world is watching him.*

SUMMARY OF CRAIG

PN: *For a number of young men and women who experience psychotic breaks and schizophrenia one can see, just prior to the onset of their disorder, heightened stress, increasing tension, and at times conflict and impasse over issues that are of concern to them (Bowers, 1974). The increased stress usually results in heightened cognitive arousal with diminished inhibitory function. This can lead to an intermingling of personal concerns and conflicts into one's thinking, to disorganization-confusion, and to impaired self-monitoring (Harrow et al., 1989; Port et al., in press). While the above models, with the heightened state of tension and stress, can be observed in a number of young people who experience psychotic breaks, they do not apply automatically to all schizophrenia patients and they do not easily fit Craig's account. It seems likely, in reaction to Craig's history, that there is not one event or issue or a clear set of issues that tipped the balance and led Craig, who presumably was already a vulnerable young man, to his psychotic break. There are still many aspects involved in the pathogenesis of schizophrenia that mental health professionals do not understand.*

Once Craig became psychotic, one can see how his delusions and altered sense of reality put him into a subjective world that in one way is quite different from the real world but contains parts that are consonant with the real world. Craig understood the hospital setting by which he was surrounded and knew who many of the doctors were. At the same time, however, Craig suggested the idea of parallel realities in which the Nazis and KKK found an image of his father sitting in an easy chair. In this sense, Craig's material is an illustration of how most psychotic patients are living partly in the real world and partly in their own delusional world, rather than being totally delusional in all aspects all day long.

Throughout Craig's illness, he continues to fight to prevent being controlled by others, by hallucinations and voices, and finally, by his own illness. While Craig is ill, he remains hopeful that somewhere inside of him is the real Craig, and eventually he will return to the real world.

REFERENCES

Andreasen, N. C., & Powers, P. S. (1974). Overinclusion thinking in mania and schizophrenia. *British Journal of Psychiatry, 125,* 452–456.

Andreasen, N. C., & Powers, P. S. (1975). Creativity and psychosis: An examination of conceptual style. *Archives of General Psychiatry, 32,* 70–73.

Benson, D. F., & Stuss, D. T. (1990). Frontal lobe influences on delusions: A clinical perspective. *Schizophrenia Bulletin, 16,* 403–411.

Bentall, R. P., Kinderman, P., & Kaney, S. (1994, March). The self, attributional processes and abnormal beliefs: Towards a model of persecutory delusions. *Behavior Research & Therapy, 32*(3), 637–646.

Bowers, M. (1974). *Retreat from sanity.* New York: Human Sciences.

Breier, A., Schrieber, J. D., Dyer, J., & Pickar, D. (1991). National Institute of Mental Health longitudinal study of chronic schizophrenia. *Archives of General Psychiatry, 48,* 236–246.

Cameron, N. (1963). *Personality development and psychopathology: A dynamic approach.* Boston: Houghton Mifflin.

Cameron, N., & Margaret, A. (1951). *Behavior pathology.* Boston: Houghton Mifflin.

Frith, C. (1995). Functional imaging and cognitive abnormalities. *The Lancet, 346,* 615–620.

Frith, C., & Corcoran, R. (1996). Exploring "theory of mind" in people with schizophrenia. *Psychological Medicine, 26,* 510–530.

Frith, C. D., & Done, D. J. (1988). Towards a neuropsychology of schizophrenia. *British Journal of Psychiatry, 153,* 437–443.

Green, M. F., Neuchterlein, K. H., Ventura, J., & Mintz, J. (1990). The temporal relationship between depressive and psychotic symptoms in recent-onset schizophrenia. *American Journal of Psychiatry, 147,* 179–182.

Harrow, M., Lanin-Kettering, I., & Miller, J. G. (1989). Impaired perspective and thought pathology in schizophrenic and psychotic disorders. *Schizophrenia Bulletin, 15,* 605–623.

Harrow, M., Lanin-Kettering, I., Prosen, M., & Miller, J. G. (1983). Disordered thinking in schizophrenia: Intermingling and loss of set. *Schizophrenia Bulletin, 9,* 354–367.

Harrow, M., MacDonald, A. W., Sands, J. R., & Silverstein, M. L. (1995). Vulnerability to delusions over time in schizophrenia, schizoaffective and bipolar and unipolar affective disorders: A multi-follow-up assessment. *Schizophrenia Bulletin, 21,* 95–109.

Harrow, M., & Miller, J. G. (1980). Schizophrenic thought disorders and impaired perspective. *Journal of Abnormal Psychology, 89,* 717–727.

Harrow, M., Rattenbury, F., & Stoll, F. (1988). Schizophrenic delusions: An analysis of their persisting of related premorbid ideas, and of three major diagnosis. In T. Oltmanns & B. Maher (Eds.), *Delusional beliefs* (pp. 184–211). New York: John Wiley and Sons.

Harrow, M., Sands, J. R., Silverstein, M., & Goldberg, J. F. (in press). Course and outcome for schizophrenia vs. other psychotic patients: A longitudinal study. *Schizophrenia Bulletin.*

Harrow, M., & Silverstein, M. (1991). The role of long-term memory (LTM) and monitoring in schizophrenia: Multiple Functions. *Behavior and Brain Sciences, 14,* 30–31.

Johnstone, E. C. (1990). What is crucial for the long-term outcome of schizophrenia? In H. Hafner & W. F. Ganttaz (Eds.), *Search for the causes of schizophrenia, Volume II.* (pp. 67–76). Berlin: Springer-Verlag.

Kaplan, K. J. (1990). Isaac and Oedipus: A reexamination of the father-son relationship. *Judaism, 39,* 73–81.

Kaplan, D., Holtzman, K., Harrow, M., & Sands, J. R. (1993, April 29–May 1). *Are the delusions of schizophrenic, schizoaffective and affectively disordered patients consistent over time? A 10-year follow-up study.* Presented at the 65th annual meeting of the Midwestern Psychological Association, Chicago, IL.

Kinderman, P., & Bentall, R. P. (1996, February). Self-discrepancies and persecutory delusions: Evidence for a model of paranoid ideation. *Journal of Abnormal Psychology, 105*(1), 106–113.

McGlashan, T. H. (1984). The Chestnut Lodge followup study: II. Long-term outcome of schizophrenia and the affective disorders. *Archives of General Psychiatry, 41,* 585–601.

Port, J., Harrow, M., Jobe, T., & Dougherty, D. (in press). Thought disorder in adolescent schizophrenics: Toward an integrative model. In L. T. Flaherty (Ed.), *Annals of Adolescent Psychiatry, Volume 21.* Hillsdale, NJ: The Analytic Press.

Tsuang, M. T., & Fleming, J. A. (1987). Long-term outcomes of schizophrenia and other psychoses. In H. Hafner, W. F. Ganttaz, & W. Janzarik (Eds.), *Search for the causes of schizophrenia* (pp. 88–97). Berlin: Springer-Verlag.

ABOUT THE AUTHORS

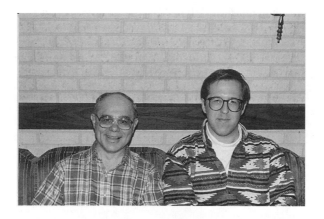

Stuart Emmons (above left) was born in west Michigan and enjoyed his youth. After graduating *cum laude,* he did further college work in three more colleges. He was in and out of four hospitals with schizophrenia from 1965 to 1969, during which time he also taught in two schools. Today Stuart reads, writes poetry, and goes out for hot tea at restaurants with friends.

Craig Geiser (above right) was born in 1959 in Holland, Michigan. Three different times he has had relapses, and he was off medication for five years. He thought he was of "the third that got better" [well], but now feels he was wrong. Divorce was equally as difficult for him as dealing with schizophrenia. Craig's son and Craig's fiancée help him look to the future.

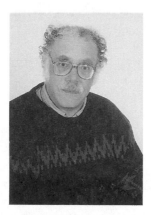

Kalman J. Kaplan, Ph.D., is Professor of Psychology at Wayne State University and Director of the Center for Suicide and Self-destructive Behaviors at Columbia-Michael Reese Hospital and Medical Center where he is an attending psychologist. Dr. Kaplan is associate editor of *The Journal of Psychology and Judaism* and on the editorial board of *Omega: The Journal of Death and Dying.* He is co-author of *The Family: The Biblical and Psychological Foundations* (1984) and *A Psychology of Hope: An Antidote to the Suicidal Pathology of Western Civilization* (1993), and is co-editor of *Jewish Approaches to Suicide, Martyrdom, and Euthanasia* (1997). Dr. Kaplan is also author of *TILT: Teaching Individuals to Live Together* (in press) and has written numerous articles and book chapters about religion and mental health, interpersonal relations, and suicide.

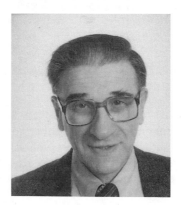

Martin Harrow, Ph.D., is a widely cited expert on schizophrenia, is Professor and Director of Psychology in the Department of Psychiatry at the University of Illinois College of Medicine, and Professor in the Department of

Psychology at the University of Illinois at Chicago. Prior to taking his current position, he was a senior faculty member at Yale University and then a professor for many years at the University of Chicago. He has engaged in extensive research on thought disorders, psychosis and long-term adjustment in schizophrenia, other psychotic disorders, and affective disorders. Dr. Harrow has published over 200 scientific papers and several books in these areas and is on the editorial board of several major scientific journals, including the *Schizophrenia Bulletin*. He has held research grants for the National Institute of Mental Health for over 20 years and is Director of the Chicago Followup Study.